Physician Relations Today: A Model for Growth

By

Carolyn Merriman, FRSA (Fellow Royal Society of Arts)
President
Corporate Health Group, LLC (CHG)
Corporate Office:
7 Brayton Meadow
East Greenwich, RI 02818
(401) 886-5588 ext. 201
(888) 334-2500 ext. 201
www.corporatehealthgroup.com
cmerriman@corporatehealthgroup.com

Kriss Barlow, RN, MBA
Senior Consultant
Corporate Health Group
Midwest Office:
651 Old Highway 35 South
Hudson, WI 54016
(715) 381-1171
888-334-2500 ext. 250
www.corporatehealthgroup.com
kbarlow@corporatehealthgroup.com

Contributing Editor:

Susan Houston Klaus
(402) 758-0827
sklaus@tconl.com

Acknowledgments

Thoughts and words are not created in a vacuum—and ours were built from longstanding personal and professional relationships. Without these learning and trusting relationships we would not have been able to develop and share our ideas on physician relations and sales strategies. We hope that all of you capture ideas, techniques and a passion for exploring physician relations and relationship sales strategies. We wish you the best.

This book could not have begun to be written without the support of our clients and their organizations. Their challenges, opportunities and willingness to innovate provided us with a wonderful laboratory. We hope we've reflected our clients' ideas, visions and models accurately. Any mistakes rest with us.

To our clients: We thank all of you for your willingness to help, listen and learn with us on this journey.

Kriss Barlow
Carolyn Merriman
September 2004

* *

At Corporate Health Group, I believe we are blessed with the best clients in the world—hats off to them. They passionately believe in the process and willingly invest their expertise in partnership with us to successfully work the model. It truly is an inspiration to work beside them.

As a group, we absolutely adhere to the adage that two—or more—heads are better than one. It goes without saying, but Carolyn and I together enjoy an unbelievable working relationship and it's that synergy and spirit of collaboration that generated our desire to write this book.

The Corporate Health Group team is a talented group of consultants and associates who have lived in the trenches. I gratefully acknowledge their support and the insights that Allison McCarthy and the team provides to the advancement of physician relations. A special credit needs to be given to the planner on our team, Kerry McCormick. She digs through data in pursuit of the full picture and helps define the plans essential to a strong physician relations framework.

Great bosses push, inspire and give you the freedom to develop your professional identity: Mike Thomas was a great boss and is very much a part of why I chose to be a marketer. And on a personal note, I'm blessed to work as I want because of loving support from my best friend and husband, Doug, and our charming Barlow Boys—Tony, Jon and Greg. While they all may believe I'm a bit work obsessed, they love me in spite of it.

Kriss Barlow

* *

To our incredible clients along the way, who believed in a boutique consulting practice and were interested in challenging the norm. To the associations and professional peers that I have been blessed to laugh, share and grow with. And most of all, to the Corporate Health Group team of consultants, especially Kriss Barlow and Ginger Schneider and support staff that I have been able to work with—sharing new ideas, success stories and a passion for excellence. A special thank you to Susan Houston Klaus who has become "my voice" and managed my writing for years.

To my grandfather who taught me that I could succeed in business and my father who encouraged me to think outside of the box and that as a woman I could do anything I set my mind to. To my mother who encouraged my creativity and challenged me to make do with whatever resources were available (soup from leftovers . . .), to my sister who challenged the left side of my brain that was underdeveloped, but loved me nonetheless.

To my two stepchildren: Gina, who grounded me in what is important in life; and Betsy, who shared a passion for being an entrepreneur and encouraged me to take big steps. To my beloved corporate cat, Razz, who served as the paperweight for all the revisions and loved to walk on the computer keys.

And most of all to my friend and husband, Brandon Melton, my partner in business and in life. I couldn't have completed this without "date nights" as incentives, quiet Sundays for writing and a respect for my work.

Carolyn Merriman

Contents

Introduction

Acme Hospital's board meeting last night left the entire executive team with a lot to think about. While each presenting member of the leadership team had worked to position their focus, activities to date and their predictions for potential revenue, the numbers just don't lie. Cardiology is down by 12 percent and Orthopedics is off as well. The sad truth is that the only area of revenue growth was in Pediatrics—and that's certainly not enough to sustain the bottom line.

There are no easy answers for declining revenue; unfortunately, the "quick fixes" of the past likely contributed to the current state. One thing's certain, however—things need to change. The organization has done a good job of managing expenses. The changes made in supply management, enhanced efficiencies and a tighter rein on overall spending have made a significant impact.

Moving forward, the board's mandate made it clear: Senior Leadership now needs to develop strategies to "grow the business." Consumer choice is alive and well and there's renewed interest in how to increase the number of patients in the key strategic service lines.

Well, we'd all seen the numbers and while we were holding our own in some geographic markets, we had substantial losses in others. The truth is that the consumers were choosing physicians who were referring to the competition. Sure, we get a few of their patients, but the majority are ending up over at St. Anywhere Hospital.

Our organization has done some things to enhance relationships with the medical staff, but even with multiple programs, there's no central strategy or focused effort. It used to be that if we provided services, the physicians would intuitively know that we expected loyalty/referrals in *exchange. That "assumed approach" didn't work all that well, so what do we need to do to get more referrals from physicians?*

The above scenario might not be a perfect match to your situation, but likely you'll recognize a little of your organization in it. The logical question for Acme Hospital to answer is, "What can we do to fix this?"

The honest answer is that there's no one magic program, process or recommendation. Across the country, healthcare systems have developed comprehensive physician strategies, encompassing joint partnerships, relationship, referral and recruitment functions, collaborative quality programs, leadership integration and more.

For many organizations, this list feels more than a little overwhelming. Isn't there something that can be done to get things started—something that will begin to bridge the credibility issues of the past, help the hospital increase the satisfaction level of the physician, and give the organization a chance to earn the referrals?

There is. Increasingly, hospitals and other healthcare organizations are finding success in creating a physician relations program. These programs are not centered on just hearing the problems of physicians; we've done that before. Rather, the focus of the new program is simple: to strengthen the physician relationship, create new business and keep current customers.

If you've picked up this book, chances are you've already recognized the need in your organization to strengthen physician relationships. Maybe you've already made the big step (at least in your head) to try something different. If so, you've already crossed the first hurdle.

In the following pages, we'll show you how to build a framework for your own physician relations program. Yes, we discuss strategy—but we also give you some step-by-step tips and techniques that are essential at the implementation level. Whether you refer to it internally as "physician relations," "referral development" or just plain "sales," it's all the same to us in this context. So you'll find that we use the words interchangeably.

Like you, we've spent lots of time in the trenches and we've seen the pitfalls and the roadblocks that make it seem that trying something new will never work. But remember one thing: there's no valor in not trying. A well-built, well-thought-out physician relations program is destined to work, despite any obstacles you encounter along the way. Yes, there will be bumps (and sometimes boulders) in the road. But we hope that the information we provide will give you the fortitude to push on and know you can make this happen.

This book is organized as logical steps in the process of building a program. We'll talk about how to determine how your program should look and how to create a business plan based on your findings. Then we'll help you examine your organization from the inside out, focusing on how to find the right people for the job, measure their on-the-job performance and compensate them.

Next, we put forth some ways to manage those bumps in the road, take the temperature of your program and make sure it's on target both qualitatively and quantitatively. We'll discuss how to grow your program once it's in place. And, finally, we let our clients speak about their own experiences, sharing advice and caveats for those involved in both new and seasoned programs.

We encourage you to use this information as a jumping-off point, rather than a how-to manual. Every organization—and its physician audience— has its quirks and set of unique circumstances. So as you make your way through the chapters, keep in mind your own organization's medical staff personality, structural needs, trust level and competitive environment.

There's no easy answer to creating the perfect program—in fact, there's no perfect program. The best ones are continually evaluating, reacting and retooling. We hope you challenge yourself to use the information in this book to create a program that's right for *your* own organization.

Chapter 1

Comparing Current Models & Assessing Your Internal Readiness

"We must plan for the future, because people who stay in the present will remain in the past."

Abraham Lincoln, 16th President of the United States

It finally happened. The leadership council has included physician relationship strategies in the strategic plan for the organization. As the Vice President of Business Development, you're charged with creating the approach and getting some results. The organization has many people working with the physicians, though no one is focused on the overall relationship. The relationship timing isn't great—the owned physicians are renegotiating contracts and the large orthopedic group is strongly considering their own surgical facility. Everyone wants action, now. Actually, they want instant magic.

Congratulations! Leadership has identified a need in your organization to re-focus on physician relationships. And while you may be eager to get a program in place, it's important to take a step back and a close look at how your organization got to this point in the first place. By doing so, you'll be better prepared to develop a working plan.

This need to shift our priorities back to physician relations has been simmering for more than a decade. The managed care revolution, and the resulting all-out worship of efficiencies above all meant that the physicians' hospital relationships often were pushed aside. With limited resources, many organizations put their eggs in one basket of managed care and contracting.

But as the tide has turned in the industry and consumers have demanded more choices, managed care has become less of a focal point in today's environment. It's time to re-evaluate all of our customers—and certainly to include the physician in this discussion.

There's healing to be done, to repair some of the feelings physicians have voiced about being treated as a commodity or a cog in the healthcare system.

A 2002 survey of physicians by the Kaiser Family Foundation found that 87 percent of respondents felt the overall morale of physicians had declined in the last five years. And 58 percent said that their own enthusiasm for practicing medicine "had lessened over the same time period." (Source: Henry J. Kaiser Family Foundation National Survey of Physicians.)

Can you blame them? Physicians today report that they feel more like a commodity than a respected player in healthcare today. While physicians say they see themselves as hospitals' main customers, the hospitals themselves often haven't been blessed with such perspective. Incredibly, physicians and hospitals often operate in their own silos, doing their jobs but rarely coming together to collaborate on the big picture.

Physicians are indeed a healthcare organization's best customers—and offer prime opportunities to create strong partnerships in what have been some shaky financial times. Getting together offers a mutually beneficial relationship that either party would be foolish to ignore.

Gradually, hospitals and healthcare systems today are coming around to realize that they and their doctors share the same goals of healing, and need to make the effort to work together to advance their purpose. And if hospital leaders need one more reason to concentrate on forging a hospital-physician partnership, they need only to look at their bottom line.

Thinking About the Physician as Customer

With its vulnerabilities and challenges, today's marketplace actually provides great opportunities to think about redefining physician relationships. Today, hospitals need physicians more than physicians need hospitals. And although people may say they want physicians to be their partners, it's more realistic (and gives you more opportunity for success) to see each physician as a *customer*.

Look at a traditional customer in any industry—retail, hospitality, banking, manufacturing, and healthcare. It doesn't matter what business you're in—your customer expects, and is entitled to, delivery of some basic rights:

- Communication
- Respect for their time and intelligence
- An effort on the part of the provider to understand what they need, want and/or desire
- A willingness to see things from their perspective, to value their insights and support their role in the process

Physician relations is no different. As a hospital or healthcare system, you owe it to your doctors—and the doctors you want to do business with—to give them the courtesy of listening to them, learning about their priorities and finding a way to create a relationship that benefits both of you, and in turn, the consumers you serve.

This chapter takes a look at the models organizations have traditionally used to varying degrees of success. And it introduces a model that we've found to be effective in virtually any situation. No matter what model you may have been using in the past, we encourage you to keep an open mind to trying something new, and exploring the possibilities of change in your organization.

"The liaison program provides the visible face for The Children's Hospital in the referring physician community to demonstrate our commitment to working collaboratively with them."

Christine M. Rhodes
Director, Physician Relations and One Call
The Children's Hospital
Denver, CO

Physician Relationship Models: An Overview

Many organizations have used a variety of approaches to reach out to physicians. As you assess what you need in your own organization, we think it pays to understand some of the most popular models and the evolution of approaches hospitals and groups have used to reach out to their peers. Maybe you recognize your efforts in one of these—or maybe you've tried pieces of several of them. Each model can work, but you need to recognize each model's strengths as well as its limitations.

What we strive to do in this chapter is to give you information to help guide you to what kind of model you want to build in your organization. In our experience, some work better than others (and we're not shy about saying so). But, in the end, it's ultimately your decision to see what works best for your organization—and for the physicians with whom you want to build relationships.

The Physician Liaison – The Regional Referral Model

This was the original 1980s model that created a systematic program for physician relationships. Based on face-to-face conversations with physicians and their staffs, it primarily targeted regional referring physicians. Liaisons were told to focus on learning about any problems physicians had in referring to the hospital. They primarily visited physicians who already referred to the hospital with the intention of learning about ways to improve service. The challenge was, in many cases, that the problems simply became too complex. In addition, time spent fixing meant field time with physicians was compromised.

Many healthcare organizations have kept this model, thinking, "If we fix your problems, we'll get more business." But the truth is, if we fix your problems we may get a chance to retain some business and work with you again—but probably won't get any more or different business from you.

If the goal is retention, and the person in the role has the power to effect internal change, this model may be a good approach. However, it isn't a way to grow new business, if that's what you're trying to do.

The Leadership Liaison – A Model for the Referral Base

This is a great concept, in theory. Back in the old days, this was how all physician relations was done. Today, there's spotty use of this model; it's generally implemented by CEOs who are good at creating strong relationships with the medical staff. In this model, Leadership is personally charged with talking with physicians and demonstrating that the organization makes physicians one of its top priorities. Unfortunately, this model targets the existing referral base and is geared to retention rather than growth. Furthermore, it can be a tough one to implement.

The physicians that your top people are talking to usually are already referring to you, so the focus is on those who are already loyal to you. And leadership may have a tendency to talk with the people they see in the hallways, or the people they feel most comfortable.

More importantly—and it's just the way it is—some people in Leadership are good leaders, but not so good at face-to-face relationship building (especially with physicians). They may be best at looking at the numbers, devising a financial plan to build the bottom line, or creating an overall strategy for the organization. And the reality is that leaders have so many demands on their time, it's hard to stay on top of this responsibility.

It's a great idea to involve Leadership in creating or strengthening relationships with physicians. But at some point, if you're interested in growing your referral base, you may want to consider transitioning to a different model or adding an approach that targets new physicians and manages the relationship consistently.

Some hospitals give their specialists the responsibility of cultivating referrals themselves, meeting with regional referring physicians to build relationships. When the models were all private practice, this was a very popular approach. Generally, physicians call on those suggested by hospital staff or those who have past relationships with their practice partners.

This can be a successful model for the very targeted purpose of building a single person's practice. There are some real challenges with long-term outcomes and hoping for a hospital "halo" from individual physicians. In addition, they may promise things on behalf of the hospital that you can't deliver. So be cautious.

You can't have a dozen different specialists all going to the same handful of primary care physicians. You'll lose the sizzle. And when that specialist gets too busy, the last thing they want to do is continue this kind of missionary work—not realizing that someone else really should continue the physician communication and field work in order to keep filling the funnel of referrals.

The Pharmaceutical Model – A Model for the Service-Line Sell

Ten years ago, service-line management became popular. And as it did, service-line leaders became more accountable for their own revenue and expenses. So they looked to a model that could help them deliver targeted results for their specialty—and found it in the same way pharmaceutical companies had.

The model assumes that the physician wants to hear about the one service that the pharmaceutical-model specialist promotes. With a multiplicity of service lines, an organization quickly could be sending 10 to 15 representatives into the field. The problem then, and one that persists today, was that physicians tell us they don't want a different vendor for each product—they want a single point of contact.

We don't support this model, primarily because it's not customer focused. But we include it as a kind of cautionary tale. Its failure to recognize the customer as the main priority, and to send out too many people to do the job of one physician relations representative, causes the organization to be seen as representing a commodity and leaves an organization vulnerable.

The Referral Development Model – A Model for Growth

We believe that building new referral business is the foundation for success. New referrals drive your ability to build your brand, enhance your services and bring new people to your organization, who in turn will tell others. Physicians who are well educated about your hospital are many times more apt to send their patients there and continue to do so.

That said; a referral development model is our pick if your organization needs a physician relations program that's focused on growth. The model puts a professional representative in the field to meet face-to-face with physicians and office staff, get an understanding of their needs and discuss their goals. Here, your physicians enjoy a single point of contact to answer questions or provide insights, create opportunities and share findings with the hospital team.

The referral development model is dialogue driven and relies on the provision of information and education about services, innovation and experience of specialty physicians and their organization's differential advantages.

This model is grounded in tracking of activity and results, and holds representatives accountable for finding new business and expanding existing business. The representative has to be in the field generally 60 to 75 percent of the time to meet the basic job responsibilities and the expectations for this position are carefully outlined in a performance standards plan.

Organizations across the country have had success with this model. Some have used it entirely for new business development. But the majority employs it to support retention and new business development.

Often, the new business initiatives focus on working with physicians who currently split their business and admit patients at other facilities. For some organizations, the new business focus is regional, and still others are targeting those physicians in geographic markets who don't admit to their hospital, but certainly are treating patients in the neighborhood who may desire your facility.

The success of this model hinges on finding the right person or people and then having a structure that allows them to focus on doing their job. It also requires clinical support from the staff and physicians on staff to advance referral relationships. And it demands the understanding and buy-in of the entire internal organization.

Our Pick for Delivering Results

If the desire of your organization is to increase referrals, the referral development model is your best option. We believe it takes some of the best of what we learned in the years and models before and provides a strong, clear focus. Because clients we work with are most often interested in new business development, this is the model we generally use as part of our consulting work. It's the model we'll be discussing throughout the rest of this book.

Why? Because it's based on a growth-oriented strategy with measurable results. This model uses well-trained people to develop a relationship that holds the opportunity for your organization to grow your referral business—and retain your current physician customers. In today's economy, this model gets high marks for its ability to develop new referrals in a cost-effective and consistent manner.

Compare and contrast the model(s) you may be using currently with the referral development model:

Physician Liaison

Structure	Generalist approach; reports to marketing or medical staff
Goal	Conversation; uncovering problems
Method	Face to face: staff and physician
Territory	Local and regional referring physicians
Expectation	Learn how to improve service
Compensation	Salary

Leadership Liaison

Structure	Calls on physicians with an established relationship. Local medical staff is categorized by specialty and/or interest
Goal	Communication
Method	Face to face
Territory	Local
Expectation	Information sharing/problem solving
Compensation	Part of the job, "other duties"

Physician Directed

Structure	Specialists implement "circuit approach" to enhance personal referral base
Goal	Awareness and referrals
Method	Face to face
Territory	Local and regional physicians who are known to practice or hospital
Expectation	Visibility = Referrals
Compensation	May be employed or private practice

Pharmaceutical

Structure	Reports to service-line leadership; may be part of other duties Targets service-specific physicians
Goal	Retention and new business development for the specific product line
Method	Face to face, emphasis on telling about the product/service
Territory	Generally defined by current service draw, competition and opportunity
Expectation	New business, retention of existing business
Compensation	Salary and incentive plan

Referral Development

Structure	Generally centralized; reports to Business Development or Marketing
Goal	New referral business
Method	Face to face: physician and office staff
Territory	Local and/or regional
Expectation	Referrals
Compensation	Salary and, often, incentive plan

What Does Your Organization Need?

It goes without saying that every organization needs to determine its unique program goals, internal commitment and marketplace as they define the type of model they desire. Yours may be a hybrid. As you do the business analysis and plan (discussed in Chapter 2), consider what's needed most. Don't rely on what's worked at different times or in different organizations. Look at what you need right now, and in the next 12 months. Then work through a model plan that fits your goals.

- Evaluate your referral data and determine changes in referral patterns.
- Do a market analysis: competition, strategy, demographics.
- Gain perceptions of your internal/external medical staff.
- Solicit Leadership's priority: Is it retention, new business, satisfaction?
- Dissect the physician's current satisfaction level. Look at local, regional groups; examine loyal "customer" vs. those who split their referrals among area hospitals.
- Look at your offering through the referring physician's eyes. What can you position that offers them a value?

Getting the Internal Team on Board

Some programs fail *not* because the models aren't good or because the people aren't doing their jobs. They fail because, with the anticipation of a "person in the field," there's also a lack of focus. Assuming you're interested in cultivating the model designed to grow referrals, the next step is to match your internal and external expectations.

To get your team on board, show them that they're an integral part of making this program happen and why it's crucial to have everyone work together.

Leadership provides that top-down support you absolutely need to create this program. They provide the assistance you'll need in creating ownership of issues by the internal team and ultimately delivering on the promise.

Operations/clinical leadership is essential for program success. They're the ones who your representative can trust to provide clinical insights. They also create a quality environment for patients and support effective follow-up with the referring physicians.

The current medical staff are your allies, the source of insight into what your organization can offer a referral physician. They're also the direct-connect for referrals once the representative gets the referring physician's interest. Work with specialists in the targeted areas to discover ways to position their expertise to outside doctors. Ask them what insights would help them in their role.

"The CEO has to be personally involved. Complete access to all data is a must for the sales director. Leadership needs to understand that this is not a quick fix; results take time."

Nancy Dugas
Healthcare Consultant
Strategy and Business Development
Shreveport, LA

There's no magic formula for achieving your goal of creating relationships with the medical staff. There's no quick fix. This is an effort business, and valuable relationships are effort driven. As your senior leadership team looks for ways to enhance physician relationships, you need to focus on learning about their goals. You'll accomplish this through interviews and discussion, and most often by delving into the strategic plan to clearly define your physician-related priorities. Next, you'll need to create a process and approach for accomplishing mini-goals along the way:

- *State your purpose.* Know your reason for embarking on a physician relations program.
- *Write a business plan.* Build a framework for the future that defines your expectations and outcomes.
- *Build a process.* Detail a systematic method to which everyone on the team will adhere.

Take a Look Inward Before You Act

Sure, there are plenty of times when Business Development has to forge ahead and "just get it done." And we wholeheartedly support this approach when there's a need to create a strategic shift. But, in the case of physician relationship building and creating an environment of trust and credibility, you need the support of Operations.

Some good old-fashioned organizational self-reflection is absolutely the order of the day. It lets you see the realities: what you need, where to start, who on the leadership team needs more time and attention to grasp the concept, and what the ultimate outcome of the program needs to be.

Resist the urge to copy what others are doing. This is one place where duplication of another's best practice might not work with your medical staff. Conduct an internal assessment, define what you need and then begin the process of creating the structure, plan and process for success.

Tips to Take Away

For those just starting out:

1. The time is right to have a planned approach for relationship building with physicians. Think of your physicians as your customers; you need to earn their business as much as you do from your consumers.
2. Define what your organization wants or needs from the relationship. Let that definition be the guiding force as your build your program.
3. Take an unflinching look at what you've done in the past to create physician relationships. Then look at what your current relationships look like. Assess what's worked and what hasn't.
4. Get internal buy-in early in the process. Spend the necessary time to explain and sell the concept. You'll need these allies all the way through.
5. Decide which type of model best suits your current conditions. Then follow it—and don't be tempted to sway from your decision.

For those growing or reorganizing their structure:

1. Re-evaluate the model and requirements in light of current and future goals.
2. Work to ensure ongoing commitment from the internal operations and leadership teams.
3. Refocus and clarify expectations. The longer you're at it, the more your tendency to grow the "other duties as assigned" and dilute the referral development initiatives.
4. Talk to your current medical staff about changing market expectations. Learn their world to develop the best model for your world.
5. Clarify where you are and where you need to be. Where you were no longer matters.

Chapter 2

Developing the Business Plan

"Have a plan. Follow the plan, and you'll be surprised how successful you can be. Most people don't have a plan. That's why it's easy to beat most folks."

Paul "Bear" Bryant, University of Alabama football coach

At Administrative Council, the CEO says, "At the seminar I attended out East last week, there was a great deal of discussion about using members of the leadership team or representatives to call on the doctors and sell them on sending more referrals. Some of them had some pretty impressive numbers."

The team all knew that when the CEO saw something he liked, the next chapter was all but written. While he would always listen to logic, supported by the numbers of course, the story had to be very compelling. He wanted to initiate a physician sales program to develop the referral base. Now, it was a matter of who would get the responsibility.

He continued, "John, I'd like the Business Development team to get this done. Work with Dr. Smith and devise a way to get City General's physician referrals up. I'll leave it to you to tell us how you want the leadership team to be involved." John knew that while the assignment was fraught with challenges, he had a coveted position—and there were so few chances to develop new programs and have an impact.

If it's possible to feel two emotions at once, you surely are—something between the excitement of knowing it's time to start building the program and the realization that *it's time to start building the program.*

When you get the assignment, it's natural to be eager to "go forth and make it happen." But, in healthcare, progress usually falls at one of two extremes. A new program in development is often analyzed, scrutinized and dissected at every level. For these programs, the energy and momentum is long gone before it even gets the green light. At the opposite end of the spectrum are the programs built almost entirely on intuition—and with limited scrutiny. Unfortunately, too many physician relations programs have fallen victim to these approaches.

If the organization is committed to the physician as a customer, and if the right person is hired, there can be successful outcomes. But, more often than not, the program is set up to fail because it lacks direction.

Ignore the importance of writing a business plan and you'll pay the price. Make no mistake: A physician relations program uses expensive resources. Without a clear focus for the approach, targets and expectations, the program can move forward—but it won't provide you with measurable outcomes to justify its expense and efforts.

For this reason, it's important to do your due diligence on the front end and ensure you've crafted a well-defined strategy. This chapter takes you through each step in the process, including identifying where market opportunities exist, developing targets for the sales effort, recognizing what it takes to generate referrals and defining how the results will be measured.

The Function of the Business Plan

The physician relations' business plan and its development process allow the leadership team to objectify the current situation. With so many people involved, each with their own agenda, the business plan is a must-have tool.

A solid plan allows you to say, "Here's where the market opportunity lies, by geography, service lines and individual physicians." It helps answer the question, "What do we think we need to move forward and begin to cultivate relationships?" Furthermore, it gives you the power you need to take a competitive stance in your marketplace.

A business plan will show you where you need to focus and where you're already doing a good job. It's designed to highlight:

- Where you're strong
- Where you're vulnerable
- Who/what/where you need to target
- If you need to expand your referral base to grow your business
- If there are opportunities simply to go deeper and wider with your existing referral base
- Which medical staff members to spend your time with
- Ideas for finding new opportunities or a better way to structure your existing methods

Maybe it reveals that you have a pretty balanced approach, and mainly need to look at your capacity issues. Or perhaps it will show a need to focus on recruitment and retain all the business you have until you're ready to look outside for new business. Ultimately, your plan should identify where you can get the best return on investment, given your current market environment.

"If you've not had sales experience, it's probably a little hard to be a believer in this kind of program. You've got to have a champion if you're going to make physician sales work in your organization. That's preferably the CEO, but certainly a champion of substantial leadership in the organization.

Without that on the front end, I think the onus rests on whoever is going to develop the plan. You need to develop a business plan that looks at the costs and returns projected; then, you need to tie it back to the strategic plan of the institution. You need to articulate how you'll measure success and what metrics you'll use. Build the business plan and show the projected return and then take that to the CEO or the champion you're trying to solicit".

Wayne Sensor
CEO
CHRISTUS Schumpert Health System
Shreveport, LA

(Editor's note: In mid-2004, Sensor assumed the CEO post for Alegent Health in Omaha, NE.)

It's a Business Plan, Not the Magna Carta

Don't feel obligated to write a thesis. That's not what your plan is about. Pull some data, summarize the results of your research and include some brief pieces of rationale. The focus here is about putting enough elements together so that you can see the big picture and move forward. If you put together a solid plan, you should achieve results that will require you to examine and redirect your plan every one to two years.

Guidelines for Developing a Comprehensive Physician Relations Business Plan

---

These are the basic elements of your plan. Generally, any business-planning format your organization uses will work just fine—as long as the process examines data at the *physician-specific level*. The more specific that element of the plan is, the more useful the results will be.

1. Analyze Your Market
    - Demographic analysis
    - Analyze current volumes
    - Payer-driven analysis
    - Physician supply and demand

2. Review Local and National Trends
    - Models and innovations in market share enhancement
    - Physician integration
    - Physician/payer and provider relationship issues

3. Conduct a Competitive Analysis
    - Profile competitors

- Market share analysis
- Current initiatives/current physician relations program

4. Analyze Your Medical Staff
   - Medical staff profile
   - Analyze physician specific data
   - Review current referral patterns
   - Review medical staff perception data
   - Evaluate current initiatives/current physician relations program
   - Create a comprehensive physician database
   - Prioritize your physicians

5. Make Recommendations
   - Identify targeted physicians
   - Identify activity volumes for staff
   - Quantify expected results
   - Financial analysis

6. Establish a Process to Move Forward
   - Timeline
   - Internal development issues
   - Communication process
   - Begin tracking results

Step 1: Analyze Your Market

To whom and where are you targeting your efforts? Your market needs to be defined according to the populations you want to serve through this program—a process that follows the general guidelines of creating a strategic plan.

First, your organization looks at the marketplace and the current business it's attracting. It may well be that you've already done this and you need only to update or fine-tune your information for the business plan.

Demographic analysis: Examine the basic demographic characteristics of your market(s) looking for any trends or projected changes. At minimum, you should examine the population by age groups and payer mix. If the data shows that your population is growing and expecting a large jump in the female childbearing age group, for example, you need to take a good look at your OB/GYN situation.

Analyze current volumes: Three years of trended data is ideal. Because most organizations track activity by service line, this is usually the easiest place to start. Examine the numbers by service-line area and ask what's been happening in these lines over the last few years. Look at what you've defined as your primary and secondary service area. Where are there significant gaps or holes in your ability to draw business from those areas?

Payer-driven analysis: At this part of the plan, there's a need to understand the organization's philosophy and approach within the payer world. A payer analysis will offer detail regarding the current payer mix, trends by payer and any significant shifts.

Physician supply and demand: Now, take the next step and look at the medical staff composition in your market. Look for gaps in specialty areas. And remember that factors such as age and political loyalties may also come into play.

Most organizations choose to do a population-based ratio analysis. This tool can be used by physician recruiters as well as providing insights for the physician relations team. It is a central component to the medical staff development plan. Each specialty is evaluated to determine whether the market as a whole has enough physicians to meet the needs of the population. This study is especially necessary if you're actively recruiting, ensuring that it's available for your planning and recruitment team.

Include any background information within the local medical staff market, especially if there have been significant changes with group consolidations, changes in practice ownership or financial upheaval. Think about the local physician marketplace: What types of things may be affecting their practice development and or overall well being of the practice?

Step 2: Review Local and National Trends

Many organizations are very interested in best practices these days. They want to identify and evaluate who's doing a program or process notably and learn from them so they can replicate the results in their local market. Beyond benchmarking, this is about recognizing the nuances of why some organizations are real winners and why others simply exist. With this current marketplace thinking, it's appropriate to detail the national trends in physician relations. This will include details on the new level of interest in these programs, the strategic "must haves" for success and the tactical difference makers evident in some of the best U.S. physician relations programs.

Beyond "best practices," look at local and national trends in physician integration, managed care and payer relations. If there are challenges in your local market and future changes the physicians have concerns about, detail that information in this section.

Step 3: Conduct a Competitive Analysis

This portion of the business plan should help you to answer the following questions about your competition:

- What service lines or geographic areas are they beating us in? And why or how?
- What's the mix and "look" of their medical staff in terms of specialty offerings, age and ownership?
- What's their market strategy and current approach for working with physicians?

Profile competitors: Profile your competitors and identify their scope of services, noting areas that they have either strengths or weaknesses. Also, consider the level of geographic coverage they have in the market. Finally, gather as much competitive intelligence as you can about their medical staff composition.

Market share analysis: Next, you should quantify their positions by reviewing market share data. This data should be viewed by total volume, service lines and patient origin if the data is available. This analysis can identify momentum in specific specialties or geographic areas that you want to investigate further. This data often sets the stage for prioritizing service lines in your plan.

Current initiatives/current physician relations program: Finally, review any information that is available about your competitors' physician relations' strategies. Learn from the experience and/or mistakes of others.

Throughout the process, keep in mind that you need to build a case to say:

> "The data indicates that we can differentiate ourselves in the market by targeting areas where our competitors have gaps— whether in their current offerings, delivery systems or physician relationships."

Step 4: Analyze Your Medical Staff

Current medical staff profile: Examine the demographics of your medical staff from every angle. Categorize your staff according to specialty, age, geography, group affiliation and level of affiliation with competitors.

Whether or not you do a full ratio analysis by specialty (the supply-and-demand analysis described above) is an individual organizational decision. At a minimum, however, a physician relations business plan does need to evaluate your own staff to clearly understand who you have, what they bring to your organization, how much longer you anticipate them practicing *and* if there's adequate capacity to grow their referrals.

Analyze physician-specific data: You should now look at detailed volume data for your own medical staff and their current referral patterns. Analyze staff members by their revenue and volume over the last three years. Look at the emerging trends; you'll begin to recognize what specialties need fewer cases to generate significant revenue. On the revenue and volume side, look at the top 10 to 20 physicians. Detail who they are, their ages, their loyalty and any changes in their production according to the trended data.

You'll find an interesting picture of how to look at capacity in order to promote by specialty. For example, if you're underserved—maybe short two physicians in Cardiology—then it may not be the right time to promote this service line.

Know where 80 percent of your physician business is coming from. We did this with one client and found that their 80 percent was coming from five physicians—one of whom was 62 years old. That's fairly revealing, and shows how the data can tell a compelling story for how you should move forward, and how quickly.

Current referral patterns: Using geographic and service line data, evaluate where the referrals come from by type of business. Again, it's important to look at trended data, evaluate market shifts or changes and provide a baseline of current referral activity.

If you don't have a list of referring physicians by name, look at your discharges by ZIP code. If you're getting a significant number of patients from certain ZIPs, dig deeper and try to determine which primary care physicians are sending referrals to your specialists.

Analyze physician market share: This is a different kind of analysis than you may routinely do. Here, you want to know where your physicians are admitting their patients. What percent are coming to your facility and which other facilities are they using. If available, this can be some of the most revealing data you will examine and will become critical in prioritizing where you should spend your efforts.

This can be a tough piece of information to find. Some organizations can call on their state to provide some great data. Others won't be so fortunate.

Review medical staff perception data: Take the pulse of your medical staff and learn what they think about you and/or your programs. If you haven't done it recently, have a study conducted by someone who will be seen by the medical staff as unbiased, or hire an outsider to do interviews to gather the current perceptions of the medical staff. While this is generally inclusive of satisfaction levels with your staff, if it's "in process" as you're developing the physician relations business plan, go ahead and take this opportunity to include some of those physicians you're targeting who currently don't refer to you.

This piece of information is very helpful for the future framing of your messages. It will let you know if you have some baggage in the market and help to tell you how you're going to need to manage it. You will also find out what you are doing well. It's just as important to continue the good as fix the bad.

Evaluate current initiatives/current physician relations program: This section should detail what your organization currently offers as part of their physician-as-customer umbrella of services. Take the time to detail all the services that are currently in place to support the medical staff in education, practice development, recruitment, call center and practice management—as well as relationship development.

If you currently have a physician relations program, detail its goals, roles and outcomes. Discuss key reasons for implementing the program, and key findings to date.

Create a comprehensive physician database: This is perhaps the most crucial activity you will perform during the development of your business plan. The creation of this database will allow you to capture historical data and serve as a base for future tracking and reporting.

You should begin by creating a spreadsheet which allows you to sort physician data by multiple variables including: age, specialty, status, group affiliation, office locations, FTE status, hospital affiliations, and several years of inpatient and outpatient volumes. As you complete other areas of your business plan, transfer any important findings to this database.

This database will serve as a resource for your physician relations program but will also be invaluable from a recruitment and strategic planning perspective.

Prioritize your physicians: Using your database, categorize each physician according to: loyalty, importance for volumes, importance for current strategies and overall priority for physician relations' activities. Determine a method for consolidating all of these factors to produce a priority level to assign to each physician. This can be as simple or as sophisticated as you like.

Step 5: Make Recommendations

Now is the time to step back from the detail and put together a recommended course of action based upon all of the information reviewed. Assuming that the data you've gathered supports the development of a physician relations program, this section should reflect which physicians you will target, what level of activity your program will strive for, what results are expected and how you will measure your success.

Identify targeted physicians: The process you completed to assign priority levels to your medical staff members will provide you with direction here.

Quantify expected results: You'll need to define a system for how you will measure your results. Typically, referrals and/or admissions by specific physicians and in aggregate are compared to pre-program volumes. These are also looked at from a revenue perspective. In order to be able to objectively evaluate your program's success, you need to be sure that your organization is prepared to collect the data you will need.

Financial analysis: Crunching the numbers is an important consideration, certainly, but there's no set-in-stone formula. Some organizations make complex forecasts for revenue and volume in their key service lines. Others work from a contribution margin model and determine the number of revenue-producing cases they hope to generate as a result of the program.

The majority of organizations start the program with a desire to create a break-even financial scenario for the first year. Often, they do this because they recognize that their internal data capture and tracking needs a serious overhaul. The result? They project their total expenses and hold the vice president in that area accountable for break-even status. If they choose that route, the business plan generally outlines the areas of potential profitability and the projected expenses.

Step 6: Establish a Process to Move Forward

If you've reached this point, take a moment to celebrate—you've certainly earned it! Now, you're ready to recommend the timeline, the approach, get started and begin measuring the results of your program.

Timeline: You'll need to establish a timeline for getting your program started. Operational considerations such as staffing, budgeting, computer systems and equipment and space needs should all be considered.

Internal development issues: With good background on who you will target and the key strategic service areas for growth, there is a need to understand what differentiates the product and how the product/service can be positioned for prospective referring physicians. Examine access and availability of specialists to get referred patients seen in a timely manner. Explore the mechanisms that are in place or needed for management of questions or issues that are raised by the prospective referring physician. Decide who the contacts will be for doing physician-to-physician meetings and what value-added services can be used to advance the relationship.

Communication process: Decisions need to be made regarding tracking and communication. This includes the development of consistent messages used by Leadership and the representatives for any key messages.

For those building a new program, there are often questions about how to communicate and promote it. Most of our clients have been more successful with a very soft launch, scheduling meetings with key staff physicians to gain their insights and having the representative attend some medical staff meetings. Other than that, we recommend no major announcement or launch.

By letting the program start soft, you'll be able to work on the processes. Besides, many physicians will assume they would be seen first—and the reality is, many won't be seen for months. In addition, many of those targeted for visits aren't currently loyal to your organization and may not be reading your communication at this point.

Begin tracking results: Try to have all of your data systems in place before implementing your program so you can have good baseline data to use for future comparison. Keep a close eye on data capture; you don't want to find out six months into your program that Admitting hasn't been capturing any referring physician information.

Take Another Look

Your business plan isn't a historical document that's destined to yellow with age. Review, refine and update the information—especially the market data that will drive your strategy—every 18 months to 2 years (yearly, if you're in a tumultuous market). If your program has been successful, your new market assessment should show some major differences from the one in your original business plan.

"A successful program must include a solid organizational strategic plan/direction, which is communicated, communicated and communicated both up and down within the organization. The sales team needs this for acknowledgement that they are doing the 'right thing' but to also feel valued in their role within the organization. It helps the representatives in their planning and execution as well as on-the-spot communication."

Judy Blauwet
Senior Vice President, Business Development
Avera McKenna Hospital & University Health System
Sioux Falls, SD

For success in this endeavor, it's absolutely critical that you get business plan buy-in from Senior Leadership including finance, data, business development, operations leadership, and the CEO. It's important to gain trust and receive feedback from particular members of this group as you start and move through the process. Like you, they're key stakeholders in the process and are affected by its outcomes—so don't leave them out of the loop. Solicit their input during program development and present them with the final plan when it is ready for implementation.

Tips to Take Away

For those just starting out:

1. Be deliberate: Take the time to create a plan that's action-oriented.
2. Step back and get creative as you endeavor to determine the current market and trends. Think about ways to understand the market by physician, even if the physician data is muddy.
3. Create time lines and expectations. While you may not have an exacting forecast, you should have clearly defined areas where growth is anticipated.
4. Use the plan to demonstrate the internal integration of other physician-focused programs and services.
5. The plan should clearly demonstrate why the approach you are recommending is the right one, spell out the rationale with the data. If you can't, rethink the strategy.

For those growing or reorganizing their structure:

1. Detail your program's current goals, roles and outcomes. Discuss key reasons for initiating the program and your key findings to date.

2. Make certain you don't manipulate the numbers or perceptions to justify your original strategy. Stay objective.

3. Recognize that data will never be perfect. If you've neglected to do a plan because your physician data was suspect, do the plan now—even if you only have six months or a year of reliable, physician-specific data.

4. Don't be tempted to take shortcuts just because you already have a program in place. You'll gain more by deliberately moving through the process and taking time to consider each step.

5. Now is your opportunity to share the plan with key people on your team. This is the time to strengthen relationships internally by giving others a chance to give their input.

Chapter 3

Structure, Staffing and Recruitment

"If you put good people in bad systems you get bad results. You have to water the flowers you want to grow."

Stephen R. Covey, author

Acme Hospital historically had assigned relationship building with physicians to clinical service-line managers as a percentage of their job accountability. While some departments did well with this initiative, most were focused on patient care or, at best, fixing and responding to physician complaints. Even the best-intended "physician relations" efforts typically fell to "telling and selling" rather than building a relationship and positioning solutions that addressed the physician's stated needs. And their infrequent and inconsistent meetings with physicians failed to generate referrals for the hospital.

Acme was rapidly losing market share and physician referrals to the competition. The organization's leadership decided to assess their strategy, approach, staff and messages that were going to physicians. This assessment provided them with the opportunity to reorganize the

physician relations approach. Once the business strategy was defined,
they started with a new organizational and staffing model, position
descriptions and a process for recruitment that would objectively evaluate
internal and external candidates.

Organizing the Function

With a plan in hand and a sign-off from Leadership, your strategy is
officially underway. The next step is to organize the function itself. You'll
be faced with several key decisions at this juncture, including determining
where to house the function, to whom and where it reports and, if
needed, whom and how to hire so you can start delivering on your
promise.

Organizing the function of your strategy requires carrying out your
commitment to treat the physician as a customer—especially important in
the details of structure, staffing and recruiting. The physician relations
representative you hire and train will be charged with taking the pulse of
the physician and obtaining information based on verbal and nonverbal
clues. He or she will continually be focused on a dialogue-based
discussion with the physician, gleaning information about the physician's
practice, their patient population and their desired outcomes.

Remember, this is a dramatically different model than the vendor who
positions a product or a service-line staff member "who tells and sells"
the offering of the month. The referral development model is all about the
physician as a customer and the strategy that kind of relationship entails.

The staff in this function serves as a representative of the organization
and its leadership—and is positioned as the "go-between," managing
critical conversations and ongoing relationships that generate trust and
ultimately referral opportunities for the organization. It's critical, then

that this group is appropriately structured to demonstrate value and implied power and access to leadership.

The staff needs to be articulate and knowledgeable on a variety of topics, including the healthcare industry (no small job in itself), the physician world, the organization's services and, most importantly, relationship selling and management. Just one misstep in the organizational model, staff or skill set can damage—sometimes beyond repair—the relationship with physicians.

Yes, it's daunting. But building an effective model and finding the right people to carry it out is critical. Build it and implement it right and referrals will come. A strong model is the organizational structure and staffing that's required to support your strategy and your desired outcomes. When it's positioned correctly in your organization, it can help you bring value to your products, services and team, and help you achieve your desired outcomes.

In this chapter we'll talk about what it takes to create a model, get others on board with it, and put it to work in finding desirable job candidates.

What Does This Position Look Like?

Structure is everything in introducing a new position. It's about determining where the physician representative's job will be housed and with what types of staff. And it's about following through on the vision of the physician as customer. While there are some recommendations for successful models, every organization needs to examine the following to best determine their structure, reporting relationship and type of recruit:

- Who in Leadership is committed to this strategy and able to provide "day-to-day" support and guidance?

- Is that person well perceived and respected within the organization and externally?
- What department can best support the strategy as it was designed? Should the staff be in Marketing, Business Development, Administration, Medical Affairs or Managed Care— or within a dedicated service-line area?
- What's the organizational culture? And how should that be reflected in the recruitment process and tools?
- Is the strategy focused on growth (new referrals) or retention? This decision will drive the type of person and skill set recruited.
- How will the organization review current representatives and/or internal candidates? What values will be placed on current knowledge in comparison to the strategy shift and their ability to match the changing methods?
- What's the organization's weakness in supporting the strategy? Is it sales, training, automation of tracking and reporting, etc? The organization may choose to recruit talent that brings skills to enhance the current weaknesses to ensure a jump-start of the strategy.
- What role will Human Resources play in the recruitment process? What's the timeline for recruitment and who else should be involved in recruitment and screening of candidates? Do tools exist to properly recruit, objectively measure candidates against the position requirements and adequately represent the position accountabilities?

Where Does the Position Live?

Your business plan, desired strategic outcome and internal assessment should identify where the position is best placed for optimum success.

In today's marketplace, some of the most successful referral development growth models today report to Business Development or

Marketing. This allows the person to represent the organization as a whole and focuses on the physician as customer in a customized approach and long-term relationship. This strategy is created from the customer perspective in, rather than the inside of the hospital out. Each representative has an assigned pool of physicians and carries a portfolio of services that's strategically defined.

Other options for reporting relationships are direct to the Chief Executive Officer or to the Medical Staff Office and Vice President of Medical Staff or Physician Services.

Build a Centralized Approach

Organizations that have lived and learned from the experience agree that it's a smart idea to "centralize" the structure. Successful teams craft a referral development model to address the customer, be more efficient and cost-effective and to help create a mechanism where relationship sales is acknowledged as a valued strategic function instead of being "10 percent miscellaneous other duties as assigned."

Centralization can take many forms, while still providing the internal service line with representation to targeted physicians *and* optimizing clinical service line staff appropriately in qualified physician meetings. A centralized structure can play an important role in training, management, database, marketing and strategy.

We've said it before, and it bears repeating: This is a dramatically different model from simply "telling and selling." To position the physician as customer, your organization needs a representative who can develop a dialogue with physicians and a level of trust that will allow them to capture information about referring physicians, their practices, their patient population and desired needs and match with solutions or opportunities within and across the continuum of the health system.

Review Your Staffing & Size Needs

In many cases, in a start-up physician relations program or small organization, this function may be staffed with one full-time dedicated staff member. In these cases, the position is a one-person show. That person may be assigned a little bit of internal sales management and infrastructure development. In order to achieve the strategic results, the primary focus of this job should be 60 to 75 percent of time spent in the field developing trusting relationships with physicians and delivering the outcomes and strategies your team has defined.

Your overall strategy may be retention, growth or a combination of both. While many programs start the position with these intentions, it's easy to slip into internal patterns of assigning this staff member to service/issue resolution, database management, marketing communications and other hospital-based initiatives. Stay true to your original plan—and keep these positions focused and accountable for referral development with their assigned physicians and/or community hospitals.

If this structure is to support a large health system or a group of hospitals or a large outreach market, your organization should identify the total target physician population you want to manage, its geographic boundaries, and the considerations and time available for field referral development. As we discuss later in this chapter, it's a numbers game. If you have high expectations for growth outcomes with a large pool of physicians, then that may well require a team of physician representatives.

Your options, then, for assigning representative responsibilities will depend on several factors:

- Geography
- Metro vs. Regional
- Specialists vs. Primary Care
- Service Line
- Pool of Targeted Physicians
- Retention vs. Growth

Each strategy and marketplace is different. And each may require a different staffing model. However, we recommend a couple of things to position your organization to referring physicians: the application of geography for efficiency and a combination of metro/outreach and specialists/primary care to ensure a well-rounded mix and portfolio representation.

Determining the Reporting Level

The position typically needs to be at some form of management level so there's peer-to-peer acknowledgement of value internally. Too low on the totem pole and they'll have to work through the pipeline to get credibility and have their message heard. Your representative needs to report high enough in the organization to have a leader who can take it upstream and protect the integrity of the strategy at the leadership level in terms of budgeting, staffing and outcomes.

Let's say the position doesn't have a boss over business development and the representative reports directly to a CEO in a small hospital. Here, the position needs to be at least at a director's level so they're a part of meetings where they can share information and learn about new products or services.

In most cases, we don't recommend a direct report to the CEO—simply because a CEO doesn't have time for day-to-day staff management. Your structure may have a dotted line to the CEO and/or access to any of Senior Leadership, but for day-to-day sales planning, management, how-tos, most positions report to a vice president or senior vice president. Regardless of reporting structure, it's still critical to involve, inform and engage Leadership.

Identify the Scope of the Assignment

The scope of the assignment is your opportunity to properly reflect upon the strategy, marketplace approach, size of targeted physician population for this strategy and desired outcomes. These answers will assist you in determining the number of FTEs needed and their focused assignments. It's important to have clarity of the outcomes desired and what it will take to accomplish them—in terms of time spent setting and conducting appointments versus in-house assignments.

This is a new and expensive resource for the organization; make sure to focus the function on measurable results that are valued at the leadership level. Many clients will make a list for this function of "must-haves" versus "nice-to-haves"—ensuring that the position focuses on the "musts." When it comes time for budgets and FTE allocations, the "nice-to-haves" often take a backseat.

As you structure this position, you'll need to do some basic math. Say you only have one person working 60 percent of the time in the field. How many hours in a 40-hour workweek? How many hours allow you to complete how many appointments with physicians and office staff? Are you asking representatives to have scheduled appointments instead of doing the vendor drop-in? How about the percentage of time spent with physicians versus office staff? And what's the total number of physicians that this person is going to be accountable for working with? How many of those physicians are frequent contacts, quarterly contacts or annual/infrequent contacts?

As you work the numbers, consider the number of hours available to the person and the number of those hours you expect the person to meet with physicians. Your answer can drive whether, *realistically*, this is a one-person, two-person or four-person function or the *realistic* size of the targeted physician pool.

Facing reality can help fine-tune the outcomes sales can deliver, versus what other kinds of mechanisms are needed to communicate with physicians. Maybe you have to shrink your pool of targeted physicians or use two people to cover the areas of greatest need—is it metro, is it the region, or a combination of both? Should the territory be split between more than one position or be one territory assigned exclusively to one representative? What activities continue to be a function of marketing communications, medical affairs, practice management or Leadership?

Five Criteria for a Smart Hire

Every action you take in developing your position criteria stems from your strategy. As you build your structure and job description, consider the must-haves for recruiting the right candidate:

1. *Professional caliber and potential.* Your new hire will be an extension of the CEO and the entire organization. So this person needs to reflect an executive level professionalism and be someone who can act and be perceived as Senior Leadership. Whether you want that or not, that's what the physician will believe. And they'll believe what you send. Your messenger creates a message that reflects back on the organization.

2. *Effective communication skills and responsiveness.* This position above all else needs to be able to listen, respond and share information in a way that gets results. An articulate, trustworthy, flexible and creative thinker is invaluable here.

3. *Knowledge of how to get things done.* It may sound simplistic, but an effective physician sales representative needs to know their own strengths and limitations, and when and how to get help. This person has to be credible and knowledgeable in a meeting while recognizing when it's time to say, "That's a great question, Dr. Smith. Let me bring Linda from our clinical area back to a meeting with you so she can talk specifically about the technology that supports this procedure."

4. *A relationship seller.* This isn't a schmoozy thing. It's the ability of your hire to be able to get on board with a dialogue-based, consultative, long-term partnership with the physician and staff—all to build a referral relationship.

5. *Independent, self-motivated personality.* The physician sales representative often is a lone wolf in an organization. Often, there's not somebody managing them who comes from the world of sales. This person doesn't mind being accountable and is driven by an inner sense of responsibility.

The Name Game

Assigning a job title to this position is something you'll want to do as you craft your job description. You may choose a title that mirrors your corporate culture and lingo, or one that connotes a certain level of leadership ("director," "senior," "coordinator"). Whichever you choose, make sure you and your team use it consistently, both in-house and in promoting the position to physicians and others in the community.

While we've provided you with a listing of job title options, the most widely used ones are Physician Representative or Physician Relations Representative, Outreach Coordinator or Physician Liaison.

Physician Sales Job Titles

1. Senior Physician Representative
2. Physician Representative
3. Physician Service Coordinator
4. Physician Communications Specialist
5. Physician Service Consultant
6. Physician Specialist
7. Physician Outreach Specialist or Coordinator
8. Physician Liaison
9. Medical Staff Coordinator
10. Medical Staff Liaison
11. Medical Staff Service Representative
12. Physician Network Coordinator
13. Physician Relations Representative
14. Physician Relations Coordinator
15. Physician Relations Specialist
16. Physician Representative
17. Hospital Services Representative
18. Regional Marketing Representative
19. Outreach Coordinator or Manager or Representative
20. Director of (Business or Market) Development
21. Director of Customer Strategy
22. Director of Client Affairs
23. Director of Cooperative Partnerships
24. Director of Cooperative Strategies

Craft the Job Description

What skills, behaviors, attitudes and attributes are you looking for in a physician representative?

Develop a job description with the key accountability areas and percentage of time allocated to them. Then, using action-oriented words, identify the desired actions, behaviors and outcomes in each category.

Create a list of required or desired attributes and skills that are important to this position. If you can, work with your human resources department to identify sample position descriptions that may already exist that are similar (service-line representatives in reference laboratory, home health, DME, occupational health). Use those as guidelines for your new position. Completing this process will also help you prepare for the interview process.

A well-rounded job description should:

- Outline the key accountabilities and functions expected of the person. Cover everything—the personality, behaviors, skills, attributes and attitudes. Invite input from physicians, Leadership, service-line staff, and other marketing peers.
- Identify the percentage of time for those key categories. Maybe that's 60 percent of time spent in direct selling (relationship management), 25 percent in account management/community and 15 percent in database, reporting and service

- Think it through. If you were talking with a candidate, physician or your CEO in a hallway conversation, could you give them the top five accountabilities and tell them what a regular day on the job would look like? If you can't do that, you and your team won't be prepared to choose a person and tell them what's expected of them.

Develop an Internal Recruitment Team

Identify who should take part in the recruitment process for this position. Consider the levels of relationships this position will impact upon—Leadership, service lines and operations areas—and make sure the right players take part.

Throughout the structure, staffing and recruitment phases, you'll need to know you can count on your team—so plan ahead to ensure:

- Leadership's commitment, understanding and involvement.
- An agreed-upon focus for this function; a clearly defined role and accountabilities.
- Human Resource's assistance in development and implementation.
- Tracking and reporting systems that integrate, or talk to, internal information systems for the purpose of managing outcomes and staff performance and compensation.

Then:

- Have Senior Leadership reconfirm the strategy, their desired outcomes and their commitment to the program. If there's a change in strategic direction, budget or focus, you can craft those changes into an agreed-upon measurement system.

- Get the organization to agree on job responsibilities and what the position needs to do to be measured as successful.
- Engage your service lines and show them that their insight is valuable to you (their buy-in and loyalty are critical to your plan's success).

Defining the Job Description

Job descriptions drive the development of a performance plan and compensation tied to business objectives. Develop your job description with clearly defined key accountabilities. Establish them in priority and value, with percentage of time and specific core duties and functional deliverables within job tasks. See Chapters 4 and 5 to learn more about performance measures and compensation design.

Job Title: Physician Services Representative

I. Selling *(60% of time)*
   A. Prospecting
   B. Marketing
   C. Communication - Customer Service Operations (Face-to-face and phone)
   D. Qualification/Closing (Phone and face-to-face)

II. Sales Process *(20% of time)*
   A. Client Account Management
   B. Reporting
   C. Communication Maintenance

III. Sales Management *(20% of time)*

Interview ranking criteria establishes the "must-haves" and "nice-to-haves"' in the physician representative position. They're the measuring stick by which you'll compare all applicants, and a way to have an apples-to-apples recruitment tool.

There is no right or wrong for the criteria—they simply need to reflect the job description and accountabilities, the organization's culture and strategic outcomes. If your culture is service oriented or represents a religious mission, then that says something about the kind of person you want.

You'll want to rank and weight the values of the criteria so each candidate can be measured objectively against the framework. The criteria should be used at every interview point, including the resume screen, telephone interview, and face-to-face and team interviews.

Clinical or Sales?

We've seen organizations be successful regardless of the person's background. If your organization is interested in using a clinically trained staff member in the physician representative position, craft interview criteria to establish their ability and comfort with selling and relationship management. During the course of the interview of a clinically trained staff member, ask questions to determine their ability to prospect for new business versus their ability to fix problems or provide customer service.

If your organization wants to recruit a staff member who has strong sales skills, make sure you're able to provide the appropriate internal orientation and training on all clinical and service-line initiatives. When you interview a sales-oriented staff member, ask questions that get at their ability to listen and learn product packaging and processes alongside of their ability to translate your services into benefit-oriented solutions that meet the physician's stated need.

If you're able to have two FTEs in this function, hire one of each so they can cross train and support each other, while also supporting internal infrastructure needs by their skill set

Image and Personality are Criteria, Too!

Think about it. You're obviously not going to hire someone who behaves inappropriately or curses during an interview. Or if a certain image is important to your organization (and it always will be!), you probably aren't going to hire someone who looks like a snake oil salesman.

But you'd be surprised how many times no one thinks about that. Then, the first time the recently hired representative goes on face-to-face appointments, the representative's direct report (or the CEO) is fielding calls about the "interesting new sales representative" who was just in the physician's office.

First impressions count. Don't discount your gut feelings during your first encounters with a job applicant. Chances are, your physician customers will have the same initial feelings as you do.

Detailing Your Criteria

Once you've defined your criteria, create a one-page sheet with a column listing of the qualities you're looking for. Next to each criterion, designate a scale from 1 to 3—with 3 being the most important. Make another column beside it with numbers from 1 to 5—those are for the candidate rankings.

Example:

Sales skills	Rank (1-3)	Weight (1-5)	Total (1-15)
Ability to think on their feet			
Sales planning			
Clinical knowledge of key product lines			
Database management and analysis			
Knowledge of healthcare			
Physician relationship selling			
Other criteria specific to your strategy and desired skill/competency set			

Next, do the math: A top score of a 3 rank and 5 weight gives you a possible total of 15 points per item. As you rank each candidate following the interview, total their score and compare it against the total possible score.

Use this tool when you screen a candidate's resume, when you interview them on the phone, when they come for a face-to-face interview and when they do a team interview. Do a separate ranking for each encounter. As the candidates are whittled down to a few, you may choose to further define your criteria based on a new group of attributes.

This model allows everyone to measure a candidate in a criteria-based methodology instead of by instinct. Try it. You'll find that, all of a sudden, you get much more objective and focused on a candidate who can meet your needs. While you might get one anomaly—like somebody really loves somebody—generally, you'll find it works time and time again. It can help you manage the "personality" and gut decisions, and will help everyone come to a team decision on the right candidate.

You've selected your criteria. Now you need to develop interview questions to get at the criteria. Questions should be behavior, scenario and attitude based. Have each candidate role play, tell stories, give examples, and demonstrate behaviors. Anybody can ace the traditional interview, but they can't hide inappropriate behaviors, a poor cultural fit or a lack of skills forever. You also need to test their ability to ask good questions.

Example:

"I'd like you to talk to me about a time when you handled a difficult, angry customer. Rather than just tell me what you did, I'd like you to role-play with me—I'm the angry customer." Act out the scene with them, having them respond and manage the situation with you.

A second question might be, "So now you're back at your office with your boss. Tell me how you explained what happened with the angry customer and what you need to do internally to get it fixed."

Keep in mind that there's no boilerplate answer. You'll need to craft your measurement of the response based on your own customer service culture and desired relationship style and approach.

By asking for behavioral and situation-based responses, you'll get at the heart of the position, their cultural personality and style—not simply determining if the person can work at a hospital and go to meetings.

Develop a group of questions that provide structure to the interview process. As you move the candidate through the process, you can probe deeper and into more behavioral Q&As with each subsequent interview. Practice this type of interview with others. And make sure you don't spend an interview talking about yourself and your organization, realizing later that you didn't learn anything about the candidate!

Collaborating with the Team

While you're narrowing your field of candidates down to the top three, schedule team interviews. Now is a good time to bring in key people who will be customers, team members or people who will need to interact with this person to interview the candidate and to see the team dynamic.

Key people may include: CEO, VP of Nursing, VP of Marketing/Business Development (if they're not the boss or haven't been a part of this process), and the Chief Medical Officer. Sometimes the CEO will interview the candidate separately, but the rest of the group could participate in a team interview.

Use the criteria-ranking sheet as your guide. But also plan to have each team member ask the candidate one or two questions so the interview stays organized and focused, and your team members stay engaged in the process. Beforehand, explain to the team how to use the ranking sheet and set a timeframe for when they have to complete it if they don't do it right away, and schedule time right after the interview to debrief while the interview is fresh in everyone's mind.

At Corporate Health Group, we create a team-ranking sheet that lists all the candidates and the same scoring categories for each. This lets us look at all three of them on one summary sheet, and make a decision objectively. Then it's easy to take the sheet back to the team, and share how all the candidates ranked. "Let's talk about how we want to proceed. Do we want to bring any candidates back in? Or are we ready to make an offer to one of these people?"

A solid recruitment plan is as important to your strategy as a marketing communications plan or an implementation plan. Here, you also need to have a timeframe and assign accountabilities. Your plan should incorporate Human Resources, Payroll, management—whatever your internal processes are for recruitment and hiring. Think through each aspect of the strategy up front. Then assign an action and timeline for each element. And figure in some time to herd the process along, so that it doesn't take nine months to recruit a person you need right now. Your due diligence can help speed the process, or at least keep it from getting bogged down.

Consider some of the smaller details in the recruitment process, and make sure to figure those in your timeline. If you're going to post internally, what's the amount of time you're required to do this? When you're posting locally, what are the deadlines for your local newspaper, journal or Web site? And when responses start coming in, who will be handling the flurry of paper?

If you're going to hire outside your market, consider where you're going to post the opening (journals, electronic venues, word of mouth), as well as the long-distance interview process and relocation expenses. Work internally to determine what is an organizational standard for a national or regional search and if that will be applicable for this position. If a standard doesn't exist and you know an extensive search is required to fill this position, then gain approval prior to posting the position to ensure that long-distance candidates are protected and your organization is prepared to relocate them should they be selected.

Recruiting from other industries means your new hire faces a learning curve. Think about your "must-have" criteria and what you're comfortable teaching your employee. Incorporate the orientation and training into your job structure.

Remember, Human Resources often isn't structured or trained to screen sales candidates. It doesn't mean they're not willing or capable, but if you haven't prepped them and given them the criteria, they may not recognize a good candidate for your particular position. .

Many of our clients will pre-screen the résumés against the established criteria and, in some instances, will conduct a preliminary phone interview. At that point, the selected candidates who pass the screening can be returned to the human resources department process for the traditional scheduling of face-to-face interviews. Let Human Resources lend their expertise to legal aspects of the process, such as reference checking and screenings.

When you've found the right person, develop a six-month plan for the introduction and training of the newly hired physician representative. Integrate key service-line leadership into the process, for orientation and training, sales planning and message development. Keeping Leadership engaged in the process and function ensures ongoing recognition of the position's value and an organization as a whole focused on agreed-upon outcomes.

Don't Forget the Details

Build some of the infrastructure *before* you hire. Sounds simple, but in your haste to get to the big picture, important details can slip through the cracks. Imagine your perfect candidate's first day on the job—an expensive body in place with no defined job to do, no structure to support them and no orientation or training in sight. It's not impressive to a new staff member who's excited about their job to find out they don't even have a desk.

Tips to Take Away

For those just starting out:

1. Use your strategy and desired outcomes to build the structure, staffing model and recruitment process and tools. This can ensure a faster implementation of the strategy and successful end outcomes. Build in a plan for managing the "current staffing model" and its integration into your proposed structure and approach.
2. If you want someone to grow the business, don't look for strong customer service and problem-solving skills.
3. Recruit someone who matches your desired outcomes and is passionate about relationship development with physicians. If you desire growth and new referrals, make sure they know how to sell and be out there all the time developing new referral opportunities. If you want retention and service, recruit someone who understands the internal mechanisms of your hospital and is tenacious about ensuring that problems are fixed.
4. Recruit someone who likes doctors and having professional dialogues that move the referral relationship forward. Believe us, we've seen it all. In one instance, we were hired to review and meet with the top candidates for a job. The very first candidate, a nurse who was the client's favorite, got behind closed doors with us and said, "I just can't stand doctors, can you?"

5. Consider gathering thoughts from your employed physicians about the qualities they value in this position. Put yourself in their shoes—their rankings may be different than yours.

For those growing or reorganizing their structure:

1. Review your strategy, business plan, desired outcomes and targeted physicians. Keep what's working. Revise what isn't.
2. Conduct an informal assessment of:
    a. Leadership and physician's perception of current physician relations
    b. Current outcomes versus desired
    c. Access, capacity and service issues
    d. Reporting relationships, communication and efficiency of structure
    e. Staff accountabilities and ability to deliver desired outcomes
3. Build a new structure, staffing model, position descriptions and recruitment tools to assist you in meeting the desired outcomes for the strategy.
4. Work with the internal team for integration and/or changes in roles and accountabilities. Then communicate the changes needed for approval and implementation.
5. Set an evaluation and measurement tool of the new model and staff—and fine-tune it as it evolves.

Chapter 4

Setting Measures and Tracking Results: The Importance of a Performance Measurement System

---

"It is no use saying, 'We are doing our best.' You have got to succeed in doing what is necessary."

Winston Churchill, British politician and prime minister

Union Hospital had tried a physician liaison program in the past, but with budget cuts and a sense that the program hadn't accomplished much they got rid of the program. With a new CEO in place, a strategic plan that indicated physicians were critical components for five of the seven initiatives, physician relations seemed like a viable—and prudent—option again.

When presented with the idea, Leadership raised its concerns about a relationship sales-oriented program, saying things like, "There's no proof . . . ", "The liaison program was nice and solved problems, but . . . ".

So the CEO created a new model—one that focused on targeted physicians using key retention and growth initiatives for measurable, accountable results. He asked the leadership team to commit to a physician relations strategy, but with the caveat that they create a business plan, sales plan and performance management system all tied to accurate tracking and reporting of the physician relations sales results.
In today's healthcare environment, the economic climate makes it imperative that new initiatives be able to demonstrate results. This has never been truer than in physician relations programs focused on growth and/or retention. While an organization may approve the resources to fund a physician relations program, its members still want to see, touch and feel the demonstrated results of the program.

To report results, you must develop a means in which to translate the organization's desired outcomes into agreed-upon measurements. When these relate to a specific function's expectations and outcomes, these are called *performance measures.* Think of them as the accountability document that will point your physician relations team in the right direction and determine their level of success.

In this chapter, we'll discuss the key steps to building a performance measurement system. We'll provide ways to apply them in the recruitment, management and evaluation of your physician representatives. If you already have some performance measures in place, there are pointers to examine and enhance the process—and ideas for bottom-line contributions.

In Chapter 5, we'll also show you how you can use it to set up a compensation plan, to motivate your representative and fulfill the goals of your organization. The two work hand in hand, so it's wise to consider the two initiatives together, even though you'll start with performance measures. Finally, in Chapter 8, we'll present methods of tracking and reporting to support the performance measures system and overall program documentation.

Performance measures, by definition, are the objectives used to quantify and define sales and relationship-building goals and objectives in your program. They're the tools that allow you to clearly define desired outcomes and how they will be measured and rewarded.

- Performance measures are a detailed list of quantifiable activities, behaviors and results—in other words, a complete synopsis of the tactics or "a day in the life" expectations for your staff member.

- They become the measures or baseline by which you measure staff and each employee's job outcomes. Each set of measures is customized to the position's accountabilities.

- When developing measures, consider the qualitative activities, behaviors and results that are desired for this position. Develop definitions of what will be measured and counted as "target" performance in these categories.

- They can serve as a benchmark from which to evaluate a single employee, a job category or an entire team.

Hospitals have been using performance measures, especially with management employees, for several years. These measurement systems have been used for individuals in new departments or services, or teams involved in launching new initiatives. In some cases, organizations are tying performance measures to annual merit or bonus programs, replacing the traditional merit pay systems.

Healthcare organizations are seeking more effective ways to track and measure the results of human and financial investments of resources in business development and marketing. Today, sales-based, physician relations programs are gaining more believers by demonstrating results. Implementing performance measures offers several benefits:

1. They establish a strategic, targeted initiative that focuses on results. This is very important if you've changed your strategic model from problem solving to new referral development as it helps you avoid paying a staff for past valued activities.
2. They prove results by being directly tied to the representative's effort and being agreed upon as appropriate measures by organizational leadership.
3. They highlight staff expectations so you can focus on keeping the business you can't afford to lose, growing business with current loyal referring physicians and growing new referrals from markets and physicians where you currently aren't getting business.
4. They are measurable tools for use in recruitment, training, performance management and if available, additional compensation for above target results.
5. Competitively, they position your organization in a different relationship model with referring physicians, presenting a win/win opportunity and benefit-oriented solutions.

Remember Union Hospital? The organization had established their strategic initiatives. They reviewed their data capabilities and established a baseline of referrals into key services, along with some outpatient service areas. Their next step was to flesh out expectations into specific goals. Each one of these steps is important to the process:

- *Select your strategic and tactical physician relations sales objectives*. Review the business plan and identify areas with the greatest opportunity to contribute to your organization's success.
- *Craft specific, measurable, attainable and results-oriented measures*. An effective plan focuses on a blend of activities and results.
- *Define each standard* in terms that indicate what counts as meeting the standard and how/when it's counted.

Translating Your Strategic Initiatives into Performance Measures

Your business plan identifies the overall organizational outcomes for physician relations. The challenge now is to translate those into key strategies and tactics that you and your team can use to get results. A performance measurement system gives you, as the manager, a formal tool for converting organizational targets to meaningful benchmarks for physician relations.

Union Hospital's strategic goals translated into overall performance goals might look like the listing below. Each would have a measurable objective assigned to it so that representative activities and results can be measured and, in the long term, the program can receive credit for the efforts of its team.

- Increase referrals into outpatient Ambulatory Surgery Center.
- Increase referrals into General Surgery through the representative's work with targeted primary care and internal medicine physicians.
- Increase cardiology referrals for cath and other related surgical areas.
- Build relationships with new physicians in the community and on staff to ensure the referral options to Union are optimized.

Process for Development

While you may begin this process on your own, recognize that this will require internal support and assistance. And while there are models in this book or within your peer group networks, be advised that performance measures for physician relations must be customized to fit your organization. You can't simply borrow them from other programs or providers.

If this is a new process and tool for your organization, you'll need to work closely with Human Resources, Information Systems, Finance and your leadership team. Together, you will establish what physician relations can and cannot do, obtain Leadership's commitment to what credit will be applied to the effort and lay the groundwork on tracking and reporting mechanisms. If you're enhancing the current process, use the leadership team as you update the physician relations strategy and assigned outcomes, and to discuss the means in determining credit for results.

Selecting Your Tactical Performance Objectives

When you've defined what desired results can be directly attributed to the physician relations effort, you then translate that into specific staff activities and results within each physician representative's assigned territory:

1) Identify how their work time is spent. How much time is dedicated to direct selling versus support and internal hospital meetings? This will set the stage for reasonable target measurements in terms of number of appointments or expected results.

2) Determine what activities staff should be measured on. Consider such elements as appointments, CMEs, grand rounds, tours and physician-to-physician meetings.

3) Review norms from relationship sales programs through articles, case studies, demonstrated benchmarks and networking. Fine-tune according to your market, the demographics and expectations.
4) Craft the definitions of the measurement and what will count to the representative's performance.

Next, develop a draft performance management model. Review this with your physician representative staff and solicit their input and thinking as to definitions, tracking process and evaluation mechanisms. Finesse the measures and make sure they continue to focus on delivering the desired organizational results.

Defining and Categorizing Your Measures:

There are three areas of measures that will reflect your organization's unique needs and expectations.

- Activities
- Behaviors
- Results

Many organizations will already have the behaviors identified as a part of current organizational annual staff review and, in some cases, overall results already built out within their current measurement systems. These can and should be considered as carryover elements as you create a combined measurement system for the physician relations staff.

Activities. These are aimed to fill your referral development or retention funnel. These activities should be a critical function of the physician representative's effort as they help to fill the funnel for long-term referral relationships. They may include, but aren't limited to:

- Face-to-face appointments
  - Physician
  - Office Staff
  - Physician-to-Physician
- Group meetings
- Tours/Grand rounds
- Openings
- Events
- CMEs

Behaviors. These usually are already developed by Human Resources (HR) and are a part of an employee's annual review, but should be included in this plan. Behaviors should encompass your organization's mission and general philosophy. Behaviors are subjective to an extent, but including them in the performance measures plan makes them measurable. Remember, you and the organization define what's acceptable behavior.

Work with Human Resources to determine the required criteria, and then incorporate these into the total measurement system. If the criteria don't exist, don't think of this as a barrier. This is your opportunity to sit down with the HR team and note the behaviors that are important to this position.

Results. This crucial piece defines the measurement expectation to attribute to the efforts. They should be customized to reflect your organization's goals. Remember, that they may also vary according to your organization's ability to track and measure the results. Here are some important areas that may be addressed (more discussion can be found in Chapter 8):

- Increased referrals by targeted service lines
- Increased referrals by targeted physicians

- Retention of referrals
- New service or facility referrals

So let's re-visit Union Hospital again. Here are some examples of how they could take the strategic focus for the physician representative and identify activities and results that their performance will be measured again:

- Increase referrals by 10 percent into the outpatient Ambulatory Surgery Center
  - Identify target physicians who will refer into the center.
  - Set face-to-face appointments with five targeted physicians each week, with 20 appointments per month focused on center referrals.
  - Develop an opener/message with some sizzle and a What's in it for Me? for the physician to refer to or operate at the center.
  - Build follow-up options to engage referring physicians with the center—they may include a tour, a meeting with the new medical director, open house, and/or a meeting with the support team.
  - Continue appointments and follow-up with physicians and their office staff every six weeks for the first 90 days. Modify the level of interest and opportunity as meetings and information-sharing progresses.
  - Track responses and referrals.

How Do You Establish Target Performance?

Most performance measurement systems use a point system to establish a value for the desired outcomes. This establishes a target expectation and value—with increased values for a staff member's ability to exceed or far exceed target performance.

For activities or results critical to the success of the physician relations program, the point system can weight the measurement with a higher point range. Some organizations will place activities and results into weighted categories of percentage of value, such as 60 to 75 percent versus a lesser category of 25 to 40 percent.

Many healthcare organizations currently use three of the five measurement levels—"meet," "exceed" and "far exceeds." Regardless of which system you use, target performance should equal "meets" as the base measurement.

Your job is to identify what target performance numbers will be for each activity, behavior and result. Most organizations will set a percentage range for each level. Another factor to include is a rank/weight of the activity or results, to ensure the staff is focusing on the most important targets. Beyond allocating the target number of appointments and percent range to "target" performance, it may be important to identify that face-to-face appointments with physicians are worth 75 percent of the value, while appointments with other staff are in the 25 percent range.

Here's an illustration for face-to-face appointments:

Standard	Percent of Target	Face-to-Face Appointments
Does not meet	85-89%	14-15/per week
Sometimes meets	90-94%	15-16/per week
Meets	95-100%	17-18/per week
Exceeds	101-105%	19-20/per week
Far Exceeds	106+	21+

The percentage will help you design their quantifiable activities and results. For example, 18 appointments per week would translate to a performance target range of 16 to 18 per week. This assignment of appointments per week depends on the size of the territory, the geographic "windshield time" and other logistical factors. Do your own reality check to make sure it's realistic in your organization, market size and time allocations.

You'll also need to review the total pool of physicians and their level of priority for contact management. Alongside that is the definition of how frequently you would like for the physician to be in contact with your representative.

An example: A priority physician might be important enough to be contacted every 6 to 8 weeks. With that math in hand, you can then determine how many 15 to 30 minute face-to-face appointments a physician representative can manage over the course of a quarter and a year by level of priority.

_____

"If your liaisons are doing their job well, you aren't going to see them. Your method of evaluating their performance is completely different than any other member of your marketing team. You can't be out in the field with them every day. So you need to have outcomes and measures that demonstrate that you're delivering on the goals and outcomes the organization is expecting, realizing you're not going to be out in the field with these people every day. They need clear direction on how they're going to be spending their time."

Donna Teach

Vice President, Marketing and Public Relations

Columbus Children's Hospital

Columbus, OH

Define Your Measurements

It's important to spend the time, painstaking as the process may be, to define each measurement. One reason is that physician relations sales is not a typical function within a healthcare organization. And it stands to reason that we should clearly define the job function and what will make that function successful. Additionally, as the manager, when it comes time for performance evaluations, your job will be much easier to compare actual performance with the desired performance if you've clearly detailed what's acceptable.

For example, a defined measurable goal may read: "A face-to-face appointment with a physician will count when it is: a) scheduled with a planned action; b) information input into database, post-meeting; c) an action initiated as a documented follow-up, such as a tour, next appointment, taking the clinician with you on an appointment, etc.; and d) re-coding the physician in the target pool."

Create quantifiable, measurable expectations. Create a checklist of questions to ask yourself as you do this:

- Can they be measured?
- What's the value of the measurement?
- What's the frequency of the measurement?
- Can you clearly define, in quantifiable and measurable terms, what meets expectations?
- Can you tie the measures into a baseline from which to grow your business?
- Do you have a sales contact database to support tracking and reporting requirements?

Automating the Measurements

In order for this process to work smoothly, you'll want the performance tracked in a database system. The automation and management of the representative's activities and results will ensure an objective measurement system. It also will establish the baseline of target performance and what counts toward the standard. Additional details about database tracking are available in Chapters 7 and 8.

Using Your Measures as a Management Tool

As we opened this chapter, we positioned the value of performance management systems as an overarching management tool. And one of the most frequent uses of performance measures is at annual review time.

It's true that your measures will provide the benchmark you need to evaluate job performance, but there's a lot more that your measures can do to help you develop, evaluate and manage the program. Stretch yourself to think about them in a different way—and you'll find that they'll be welcome assets in moving your program forward.

Your performance measures can help in:

- Setting the stage to clearly communicate expectations.
- Supporting field observation.
- Implementing a data/measures review.
- Conducting daily, weekly, monthly reviews of performance.
- Building and managing the training and development of each staff member.

Recruitment

Performance measures give you an opportunity to translate the business outcomes into a person's specific accountabilities. It's an excellent exercise for you and your leadership team to use before you start the recruiting process. Determine the skills, competencies and attributes the desired candidate should bring to this position. Clearly define the "must-haves" versus the "nice-to-haves."

Use the performance measures to flesh out behavior-based interview questions to help you and your team rate their ability to meet your desired skill and competency levels. This also allows you a way to ensure that candidates are well aware of the fieldwork and direct selling requirements of the position.

Staff Management

After you and the leadership team agree on the performance measures, it's important to enter them into a database—creating one set of measures for each physician representative. This will give staff and management a way to monitor ongoing activities and results. Evaluate each measurable component at least quarterly and have an agreed-upon plan of action to address any deficiencies and/or revisions of the measures based on organizational and market changes.

Use this tool proactively throughout the year. You'll encounter fewer staff accountability surprises, and you'll see an increase in their performance results.

Training and Development

As you evaluate your staff members, use the performance tool as a mechanism to share your plans for ongoing staff training and development. This may be offered as a way to enhance and develop their skills or to address a skill/competency issue identified through your review.

Conduct a staff orientation about how to use the performance measurement system, the tracking and the reporting tool that supports this process. If pay is attached to the measures, make sure to clearly define how and when it's impacted.

Field Observation

The manager should go out in the field with their representative at least once per quarter. Use the performance measures system as a summary evaluation during the "ride along." It will help assist in observation and training, and in development recommendations. After your quarterly observation, use what you've culled to fine-tune your strategy. Share with your team the kind of information that's being collected in field visits—such as market intelligence and physician feedback.

Annual Review and Evaluation

It's standard operating procedure for a healthcare organization to annually review and evaluate their staff. In many cases, the organizational annual criteria or merit review elements dovetail with the overall performance measures plan. Some organizations have the representative opt out of the hospital merit review program in exchange for the performance measurement plan—this is especially true if there's additional compensation offered beyond the annual merit pay system.

Promotion and/or Change in Objectives

Your program's goals and objectives will change and evolve; it's part of a healthy organization. When they do, make sure to evaluate those of your performance measurement system, as well. Make sure they're staying consistent with your desired outcomes and the detailed activities and results match.

Some organizations will also identify what skills or outcomes are critical to advance a person in their position, from physician representative to senior physician representative to field managers. If this is the case, again, take time to clearly define and have everyone agree on a set of performance measures.

The first round for a new physician relations program should focus on performance measures for a six-month probationary period. This will allow for the staff training and exposure to the position alongside capturing enhanced market intelligence about the targeted physicians.

After that, review and update your performance measures regularly. Make sure you revisit them yearly, or more often if necessary. As your organizational strategy, budgets and strategic plan change, so should your measurement system.

Things do change—markets, opportunities and desired results. If you're no longer able to grow Cardiac because you're waiting for surgeon recruitment, your performance measures may need to focus on oncology referrals or other services critical to the organization's success.

Words to the Wise

- Make sure the performance measures are designed to focus the staff members on achieving the results they are accountable for.

- Measure what this person can be accountable for and avoid conflicting roles. They may capture complaints and document the information for the operations team, but it's unreasonable to hold them accountable for customer service and issue resolution, if they're primarily responsible for growth of referrals and new business into the organization.

- Make sure to discuss with the representatives what's acceptable and not in terms of activities and desired results. They need to understand their assigned targets, definitions of what is measured as success and their role in achieving the overall assigned targets.

- Look at the mix of responsibilities the representative is responsible for and weigh the jobs. Sitting in on an internal management meeting may not be as important to your overall goals as making a certain number of referral development calls in a two-week period.

- Make sure your performance measures bring order, not cause chaos. Take care to create a mix that focuses on the right accounts and coordinated customer management.

Tips to Take Away

For those just starting out:

1. Craft a management tool to confirm your organization's objectives and the measurements of success that are unique to your goals and mission.
2. Review the business plan, targeted physician pool and desired outcomes and convert into quantifiable "target" measurements.
3. Translate the objectives into key performance categories: activities and results. Assign weight/value to each and build definitions of how you'll "know" the staff member accomplished desired standard.
4. As part of your management plan, use the performance measures tool to assist in recruitment, planning and staff evaluation.

5. Allow flexibility in your measurement system. As you adapt strategy and acquire marketing intelligence, you can adjust your strategy and tactics.

For those growing or reorganizing their structure:

1. Revisit organizational strategy and physician relations business plan. Ramp up and tighten the staff's performance measures on your desired measurable outcomes.
2. Design the definitions of activities and results to ensure staff focus and outcomes.
3. Build your measurement system with an eye to enhanced staff management.
4. Ensure efficient management of performance, development and compensation by dovetailing performance measurement systems into the tracking and reporting systems. This allows for staff self-management, growth and development and customized reporting internally.
5. Grow your program by adding field observation, and address your staff's training and development needs.

Chapter 5

Building an Effective, Equitable Compensation Package

"If you pick the right people and give them the opportunity to spread their wings—and put compensation as a carrier behind it—you almost don't have to manage them."

Jack Welch, former General Electric CEO

Saint Everywhere Hospital had implemented a successful physician relations program several years ago. They had demonstrated results in terms of physician satisfaction and loyalty alongside of increased referral volumes to key specialties.

Susan, their representative, was respected by the physicians and Leadership and enjoyed her work. Over the holidays, Susan was approached by a medical sales organization with a job offer she couldn't ignore. With regret, she decided she needed to take this career opportunity that provided an increased base salary, incentive compensation and a car.

Saint Everywhere was devastated—they had to revisit their strategy, physician expectations for their representative and devise an approach to recruit the right talent and to retain the talent in the future.

Compensation, and how it's computed and allocated, is always a big consideration in any organization. While organizations have a salary compensation structure, positions such as these (physician relations) typically do not fall within the norm. It's important to carefully consider the exposure, credibility and value these positions will bring to the organization alongside of the financial contribution through their efforts and determine the base salary level commensurate with their skills and accountabilities.

Beyond the base salary, equity (internal and external) consideration should be given to performance or incentive pay for this position's additional sales results generating new or increased referral volumes for the organization.

If there's one thing we know for sure about human behavior, it's that we get what we reward.

The process of creating a compensation program goes hand in glove with developing performance objectives. As you work toward structuring a pay package for your physician sales representative, first ask yourself these questions:

1. What is the compensation philosophy in my organization?
2. What data sources do we use to establish externally competitive and internally equitable base salary ranges?
3. How do we accommodate an internal candidate for this position, especially if they are a nurse or long-term employee

4. Will our organization be willing to provide performance-based or variable pay? Or are we only authorized to give annual merit pay, and is that adequate compensation for the types of results we are seeking as contribution to the organization's bottom line?

5. Do we have an employee retention strategy—and how does that apply to the physician representative position?

Traditionally, employees in a hospital setting—particularly in a not-for-profit environment—receive a base salary, with no performance-based pay, incentive or bonus. But with increased competition in the medical marketplace and the need to reward performance, a growing number of healthcare organizations are using performance-based pay (merit or incentive) for physician relations representatives when they accomplish objectives especially at levels that are above and beyond baseline or target expectations.

Though you may have traditionally considered this decision one of the stickier ones in creating your program, it doesn't need to be—and really shouldn't be. There are plenty of resources and expert information available to help you, both inside and outside your organization. As you work through the process, seek out the assistance you need, and make sure your proposed package has the blessing of your organization's leadership and is done in partnership with Human Resources.

This chapter discusses the types of compensation and outlines the steps for structuring a base salary. You'll also find some rule-of-thumb information and industry resource contact data that will help guide you as you work the numbers.

What's Considered Compensation?

Compensation is the payment of funds to staff based upon their internal and external market-based value. Incentive compensation is monies paid for specific activities or results that are measurable and contribute to the organization's success. Components of compensation can be:

- Base Salary
- Benefits
- Perquisites
- Incentives
- Merit
- Performance-Based Pay
- Commission
- Bonus
- Success Sharing
- Gain Sharing

While it's true that some organizations don't allow incentive compensation, many do allow annual merit pay. If you're unable to provide incentives at this point, you should at least incorporate an annual merit pay program. Within that model, include physician relations performance activities and results to set the stage with the organization's leadership about key measurable results that might be components of a future incentive pay model.

Examine the Culture of Your Organization

Arriving at the right pay program for your physician relations staff and management is a step-by-step process that must be developed within the context of your organizational and corporate culture.

- Does the organization want instant results, or can it tolerate a longer sales cycle that focuses on relationship building with key referrers?
- Who will be accountable for service and delivery of the product?
- Has your organization used performance-based merit, variable or incentive pay before? If so, was it successful or were there issues that need to be addressed?
- Does the culture reward performance when it contributes to success? How does management perceive this?
- Do you have the ability to track, measure and report on sales results?
- Do you have leadership support and Human Resources' assistance in developing and managing a compensation program for physician relations?

External Equity

Whether the candidate is selected from within the organization or recruited from the outside, healthcare organizations should evaluate external market equity to ensure these positions are paid fairly and competitively. Key industries to measure these positions against are:

- Pharmacy
- Retail
- Services
- Financial
- Insurance
- Healthcare
- Sales

Determine the Type of Compensation

If you're starting a physician relations program, or if you currently have a program and are enhancing it to be more growth oriented, you need to consider how you're going to pay and reward the staff for the work they do. How do you arrive at a fair and equitable salary? How do you support the talent you've hired?

To start, think in terms of base salary and variable pay plus expenses:

Base salary, which usually comprises between 50 to 75 percent of the total compensation package, should represent core position accountabilities and reflect internal and external equity. Most healthcare organizations aim to recruit between the minimum and the mid-point of the base salary range or have established a target-hiring percentile within the range. Conditions need to be in place for annual market adjustments.

Partner with Human Resources in establishing your base pay range. If your organization is willing to utilize a performance-based pay system, develop a budget for payouts according to results. Establish the ceiling or cap on what will be offered for total payout ("exceeds" performance) and what is payout for target or expected performance.

Your compensation should also include expenses. Examples of reimbursement are:

- Current federal mileage rate
- Rental car contingent upon length of trip or size of geographic territory (for instance across state lines)
- Fleet car owned by hospital
- Car allowance approximating monthly car payment. This can either be grossed up for taxes or a flat dollar amount. Car allowances range from $250 to $750 per month.
- Provision of credit card for gas/maintenance
- Reimbursement for direct expenses related to the job as approved by management
- Computer software
- Cell phone
- Meals
- Travel

Variable pay—dollars offered beyond the base salary—can be comprised of merit pay, performance-based pay, commission and/or bonus. For physician relations positions, we recommend that you tie performance-based systems to measurable performance objectives and organizational results. Variable pay should support the desired strategic and operational initiatives of the organization in terms of revenues and volumes.

Performance-Based Pay and Its Variations

Performance-based pay can take the form of a true merit-pay program where the healthcare organization will establish a pay increase range annually. Currently, the range has been from a 0 percent to 7 percent annual increase in pay depending upon the financial performance of the organization.

A *variable or incentive compensation plan* recognizes and rewards either individual or team performance. It may be paid out monthly, quarterly, semi-annually or annually. In order to be more closely tied to results monthly or quarterly payouts are recommended. This form of pay—tied to activity and results—usually ranges from 0 to 25 percent of the base pay of the timeframe for payout. Performance standards need to be difficult enough that target performance is a stretch objective, but is still achievable.

Team performance-based payouts usually are based upon the results of the team against measurable results. Payouts can also range from 0 to 25 percent of the annual base pay for each team member. Another team payout structure is to assign a dollar amount to each measure; if the team hits only one of them, they get only that amount—but aren't penalized by other measures not being accomplished.

Stretch and "Blitz" Bonus

A stretch bonus is designed to encourage a representative or team to far exceed goals (e.g., 110 percent of budgeted revenue). This format usually covers one to three goals, such as revenue, volumes and/or and customer satisfaction.

The blitz bonus focuses on key strategic initiatives or service line launches over a limited timeframe. It may focus on a special event, such as a grand opening. Over a 90-day period, for example, the representative focuses on generating tours, new appointments, or referrals by the physicians to your center. Keep in mind that when you promote a blitz bonus and have your representative focus on these extra dollars, other initiatives may slow.

"You can't afford to have staff turnover in these positions. They build trust and credibility with physicians and you don't want to have to keep recruiting, training and reintroducing a new rep to your referring physicians. They'll begin to wonder what's going on over there, so it's really important to get long-term employees because of the relationships. And you're going to have to pay them well in order to get that. That's the reason you want a higher salary base. You also want a higher level of professional representing your system to a very important customer—the referring physician.

At first, my HR department was hesitant to increase salaries for this position. They said, 'Well, they don't really sell' because they don't get a contract signed by the physician. But I was able to compare the position with other salespeople in our organization, like a medical lab service and a home care staff member. I think it's key to look at their range. Look at what you're paying others. It's really about keeping them."

Kathy Dean
Associate Vice President, Marketing
Geisinger Health System
Danville, PA

- Corporate Health Group research, as of this writing, finds the national base salary for physician relations representatives averaging between $48,000 and $95,000 (on the higher end for those with experience and clinical backgrounds).
- In larger cities, on the coasts or for large health systems, base pay averages closer to $65,000 to $95,000.
- Performance pay averages 12.5 to 17 percent annually with stretch bonus payouts of up to $10,000 per initiative.
- A high-level manager of a large function may receive base pay of $75,000 to $125,000 per year, plus performance pay.

Where to Find the Data

These management and compensation firms can help with background and benchmarks as you compare and prepare salary information:

CompData
www.compdatasurvey.com
800-300-9570

Sullivan, Cotter and Associates
www.sullivancotter.com
212-332-3288

Hay Group
www.haygroup.com
215-861-2000

Towers Perrin
www.towersperrin.com
212-309-3400

Hewitt Associates
www.hewitt.com
847-295-5000

Watson-Wyatt
www.watsonwyatt.com
202-715-7000

1. *Write a job description.*

   Develop job descriptions with clearly defined key accountabilities. Establish them in priority and value, with percentage of time and specific core duties and functional deliverables within job tasks. Job descriptions drive the development of a performance plan and compensation tied to business objectives.

2. *Be crystal clear in defining measurable results.*

   Look at the activities it will take to generate business. Clearly define and quantify what you want your staff to accomplish.

3. *Examine the internal market value within the organization.*

   Are there any other comparable positions currently within the organization? What title and pay level are they and what are their key job functions and accountabilities? Even if the comparable position is not an exact match, you can still use it as a comparison. Home health, pharmacy, durable medical equipment, rehabilitation, occupational health sales, or cardiac service line specialists share some of the job accountabilities.

4. *Compare the external market value within your community and/or region.*

What would it take in today's market to fill your position or recruit a person from another employer in your community? What is the market paying? Compare other intangible service-based industries such as hotels, banking, financial services, insurance, managed care and other healthcare and non-profits. Unfortunately, the pharmaceutical industry is not a good comparison; their plans are typically too rich for our budgets.

5. *Conduct salary surveys.*

Review compensation studies used by your own human resources department to provide more value to your analysis and gauge how it is perceived within your organization. Look to benefits and compensation-consulting firms that publish annual reports—such as Hay, Hewitt, Mercer, Towers-Perrin, Watson-Wyatt—for help in setting the position's market range and value. If the exact job title isn't listed, look to home health, customer service representative, account manager, sales.

6. *Determine the value of sales by senior management.*

In many successful organizations referral development (sales) will be directly tied to the organization's overall strategic initiatives. Sales results must be "trackable" and measurable. In order to make a case for compensation, results must contribute to overall organizational success. Be specific about what you want the position to achieve and what you'll reward.

7.   *Review the organizational chart.*

Where the position lands on the organizational chart and its reporting structure impacts compensation and value. What level must physician representatives be at for maximum power and influence? Sales staff within a hospital organization typically report to the Vice President of Business Development, or Marketing. Understand that if the representatives are not placed appropriately within the organization, they may not be valued internally or by their key customers.

What if Your Organization Doesn't "Do" a Compensation Package?

We recognize that some healthcare organizations simply don't provide additional monetary compensation beyond base pay. But that doesn't mean you can't establish some ways to reward and recognize their contributions. Consider gift cards, catalog points, conferences/training or paid time off. And find out what other departments do in terms of employee reward and recognition, you may be able to join their already developed program or pilot a model together.

It's true that creating a compensation plan that fits your program's goals isn't a one-step process. But taking the time to evaluate what you need in your plan will help you support your recruitment efforts, focus on enhanced staff performance and develop a process for recognizing above-target outcomes.

Keep in mind that, in some cases, this kind of compensation may be a new, probably foreign, idea for Human Resources and other departments in your organization. They'll become more comfortable if you come to them with examples of other healthcare organizations or similar companies' pay, performance and bonus structures. You may be forging new ground here, but you'll need to do your homework.

Tips to Take Away

For those just starting out:

1. A compensation plan that matches the strategic focus and encourages staff members with pay tied to results will ensure your organization's accomplishment of desired outcomes.
2. Make sure your compensation plan and incentives are designed as market sensitive, internally and externally. Use your human resources department or external consultants to research the market, your own organization and the types of positions/candidates who will be applying. Make sure to assess what kinds of pay programs currently exist within your organization in such departments as laboratory, pharmacy, home health, DME, occupational health, rehabilitation to name a few.
3. Build a compensation plan that's tied to the performance and measurement results.
4. Review annually for market competitiveness.
5. Remember, it costs more to start over than to keep talent that's performing well.

For those growing or reorganizing their structure:

1. If you already have a compensation plan, review it to make sure it is in alignment with your business plan, key strategic outcomes and performance measures. If it isn't, update the compensation plan.
2. If you have a well-designed base salary compensation design, but do not currently have incentives, build a plan for your organization to assess and model incentives.
3. If this year's plan is to add incentives, the optimum model ties them to measurable performance standards that reflect desired activities and results.
4. If you're not able to offer a comprehensive incentive program, work to develop short-term project-based bonus or non-monetary rewards to allow the program to recognize achievements beyond target performance.
5. To ensure staff retention, seek car allowances, conference or training options, "senior" title status and other perks to acknowledge tenure and staff success within the program.

Chapter 6

Sales and Staff Management

"It is more difficult to move an object that is completely at rest than it is to guide one that is already in motion."

Gene Griessman, author and professional speaker

Bill Smith had been doing physician liaison visits as part of his job for the past several years. The office staff knew him well and looked forward to his visits, a box of doughnuts from the local bakery and a warm smile. While Bill seldom met with the physicians, he had a good relationship with the office staff and his boss, the VP of the Medical Staff, felt this kind of link was important.

But Business Development is talking more and more about a physician relations program—leaving Bill and his VP a little puzzled. After all, Bill wasn't doing a bad job, was he? And though no one seemed to know or appreciate it internally, Bill felt like he had done everything that was asked of him. Frankly, he's frustrated hearing that the proposed program is getting lots of positive attention and enthusiasm for something he perceived he already was doing.

For many organizations that have a "Bill" in place, there may be a certain level of acceptance—but also a lack of understanding about how that position can be developed to create more than just recognition and appreciation. For other organizations that at one time had this type of program in place, they were forced to discontinue the program when the financial screws tightened.

As we look to create a growth-oriented model that can create business opportunities in the present market, there's a strong need for clarity regarding the role and expectations. Whether an old program is re-tooled or a new program is developed, leaders need to define the process, expectations and outcomes for success.

This chapter covers some of the infrastructure areas encompassed in setting up or managing a physician relations program. Each section provides insights and action steps to help the new or mature program advance their organizational efforts in running a physician relations sales operation. While some of these topics may shed light on any healthcare management situation, we've found that a lot of them have emerged due to the newness or "non-fit" of sales into a healthcare organization's culture. We hope this chapter helps you pre-empt those issues and/or properly build your infrastructure to support the desired outcomes.

Optimizing Your Program's Value

Many people who work in healthcare believe that if you do the right thing—and do the best you can for patients—then the organization will reward you. It's an admirable philosophy, but the reality is that many good programs have been dissolved or inadequately funded because there was no internal recognition of the value.

It's not the job of Leadership to find out how effective the physician relations program is, or can be. It's the job of the physician relations team to consistently demonstrate that value. Whether you call it "internal communication," "political positioning" or "internal sales," the essence is still the same: There has to be a plan for communicating the value of the program to Senior Leadership.

Don't Get Complacent

The internal sales process begins with program development and must receive ongoing, planned attention. A word of caution here: There are times when mature programs begin to assume that there is ongoing interest and recognition of value. They may lose some of the discipline for consistent internal communication that was employed at the onset. Complacency creates a dangerous scenario. And as the program matures, there will be different measures, messages and even more retention work—so internal positioning will require dedicated, consistent attention.

Developing the Program

For many business development and/or marketing leaders, there's an assumption that the leadership team is interested in having you "just make it happen"—but with their limited input. The business development team does the research, creates the business plan and comes back with a recommendation.

While this works for most programs, certainly, this isn't the most effective way to develop a physician relations program. That's primarily because of the intricate nature of the physician–hospital relationship, but also because of the number of stakeholders involved at the senior level. Our recommendation: Create a defined approach for involving medical staff and key members of the leadership team *at the onset.*

If you're part of a large group practice interested in developing a physician relations model, the same rules apply. There should be a task force of senior partners with at least one representative physician newcomer and the office manager all working in concert to create the program's infrastructure. This model optimizes the different staff and physician perspectives and enhances the positioning to their desired referral partners.

Dealing with Internal Power Struggles

In most healthcare organizations, the physician relations program has a variety of customers. The most obvious is the referring physician—an external customer—whom the representative works with to provide information and resources in hopes of generating business opportunities.

Internally, there are also multiple customer groups. Each has their own set of program expectations, assumptions about who should provide what, perceptions of their role in the process and issues related to who's getting credit for achieving strategic goals within the organization.

While each organization needs to create their own list of customers, often it will include the CEO, COO and CFO, VP/Chief of Medical Affairs and key service-line leaders. Traditionally, many of these individuals have personally been charged with some aspect of making relationships with physicians fruitful for the organization.

As the new model evolves, it's critical to get internal customer buy-in, understand what role they hope to play in the future model and how they expect to be involved—and most importantly, what they expect to measure in terms of outcomes.

Lots of existing programs find themselves coming back to this step and this process because there wasn't a strong emphasis on this accountability piece when the model was first created. Too often, each department has continued with its own agenda, leaving the model, and the physician relationship vulnerable. There are too many agendas, too many messengers and too little clarity of who will manage the relationships. If you find you're spending more than an hour a week managing internal turf wars, it may be wise to go back through the process and, with the support of the CEO, redefine the program expectations and clarify the roles.

Creating an Internal Communication Plan

Internal turf wars are often the result of a department's concerns about what might be said about them, what might be promised on their behalf or perhaps what problems the physician will air related to their process or delivery. In other words, they are nervous about having someone else involved in the relationship. This is never truer than when the service-line leadership is asked to give up his or her own representative and switch to a generalist model with one representative for the entire organization. However, forewarned is forearmed. Knowledge and early involvement are powerful tools in managing the anxiety of the internal team. It is the job of the physician relations team, especially the leadership of the team to create an internal communication and involvement strategy to manage this and assure the service lines that you are with them—not against them.

1. *Determine who needs to be in the loop for which elements of information.*

   When developing internal reports and updates detailing the physician relations effort, consider the type and depth of information the internal team wants or needs. Some people will need to know only the general topics you're discussing. Some may need to see market intelligence. Some may need to understand the impact of competitive strategies on your referral base. Some may need to hear issues or concerns related to some aspect of your service and delivery. The CEO and Vice President of Medical Affairs will likely need to see and hear it all.

2. *Establish a format.*

   The report on physician relations activity and results should be consistent in format—no longer than a written or e-mailed one-page version. It should be brief and prepared regularly. Consider something that will make it stand out from other reports: Print it on blue paper or use a unique header, for example. The format may include three to five sections with specific areas of content covered in each report.

3. *Create a template so you can easily customize the content.*

    If you're using an automated database, look for ways to customize your drop-down menus to simplify and quantify your findings.

    Areas that may be included—again, depending on the recipient—are:

    - Activity, including total numbers of visits and with whom
    - Events
    - Key services that are being positioned and their frequency
    - Market intelligence
    - Positive comments
    - Service issues and what's been done to address them to date
    - Targets for the next month
    - Results, provided quarterly

    There are times where an anecdotal story is all you have to illustrate a point. However, if possible work to have all report content verifiable. Provide positives; if they're not providing them, ask for them (this is especially true for the service-line leaders). Use bullets and short sentences to convey the trends.

4. *Aim for continuous improvement.*

    Program leaders will need to test the effectiveness of the content and format at six-month intervals to see if the report is serving its purpose. Rather than saying, "What else would you like to see in our reports?" the program leader should try to utilize yes/no or ranking questions to determine the value of key report topics and identify future desired items.

Manage the time and effort the field staff spends on this process. They need to have involvement, but not to the extent that it becomes a burden or detracts from their time in the field.

Building Internal Communication—Beyond the Report

Beyond reporting the field findings and outcomes of the program, the physician relations team needs to connect with the internal team (comprised of Operations, clinical and key support staff). Most notably, they need to work with Operations to learn differential advantages of the services provided. By collaborating with the clinical leadership, the physician relations staff will be able to learn the features and capabilities of different service lines and supporting specialists. What's more, there's an opportunity to better understand the type of information that a referring physician might be interested in learning.

The operations team can often provide insights into the patterns and styles of current referring physicians. For the component of your retention-driven program, they'll offer valuable implementation and user insights.

Clinical experts also understand the nuances of their services, and which of those nuances would have more appeal by the different specialty types of referring physicians. Again, take the time to do this research with the internal team and you'll give your program an edge.

The internal team that feels more a part of the physician relations strategy is much more likely to be responsive when you uncover unmet needs. As with all relationship building, it's best to start the process before you have an issue or problem. The physician relations team needs to lead this initiative and not expect that the operations people will drive the communication effort.

Keeping the Internal Team Involved

Repeat after us: "It's an absolute no-no to have your physician relations team involved in all the meetings where they may be good contributors." Because their focus should be creating relationships in the field, the meetings they attend should be few and far between. Schedule regular team meetings on Monday mornings or Friday afternoons when it's not optimal field time.

Having said that, how do you ensure the representative is connected and keeping a pulse on the internal workings of the organization? This is a key responsibility of the leader responsible for overseeing the program. Represent the field team at internal meetings, give the team credit and discuss what they're learning. In addition, make sure to document other learnings that may impact the team's role and then design a mechanism for communicating this to the team.

Create a mechanism—likely including some type of recognition with it—for encouraging internal staff and Leadership to communicate physician market intelligence to the program staff. In addition, there needs to be work done with the internal team to craft an organizational model of the physician-as-customer. Have the internal staff develop processes and protocols in key access points of the organization, such as scheduling, medical records, medical staff and issues/complaints that enhance the level of service delivery.

Encourage the team to actively recognize that the organization needs physicians to admit patients to be successful. Nurture the philosophy that it's everyone's job to provide a satisfactory experience for each physician every time they have the opportunity to work with your organization

If your facility is using the physician relations staff member to represent the organization as a whole (generalist model), optimize the internal clinical and operations team members as depth to the selling process. The generalist can initiate the physician relationship, determine their needs and qualify them for a meeting when appropriate with clinical, administrative or specialist teams. The generalist will then identify appropriate follow-up from the meeting and continue to manage the relationship with the physician on behalf of the organization.

Provide preparation and insight to the internal team members to ensure a successful visit with the physician. This is an excellent way for the internal operational staff to "see, touch and feel" relationship sales, participate in a valuable team selling experience and be involved at an appropriate level with the physician as a customer of the organization.

Working Through Operational Problems

While the focus of physician relations is on relationship building through education and communication, there are times when the physician communicates a service problem to the physician relations representative, regardless of the model employed. Here, the representative can't take sides. Rather, their role is to gather background on the issue, let the physician know that the internal team takes physician concerns very seriously and convey that the representative will want the opportunity to personally investigate and respond to the physician.

Problem management does require a systematic process and a point person so that well-intended people have a defined approach and nothing slips through the cracks. The key in issue resolution is to communicate that you *heard* the issue. Whether you have an immediate fix or not, the physician needs to hear that you listened, shared internally and are looking at ways to respond.

Issue resolution can be defined as a quality process for the management of issues, concerns, complaints or communication needs. Many organizations have an issue or satisfaction process in place for patients and physicians and can enhance the current system to embrace the information captured through the physician relations program.

Following Through—Key Steps to the Issue Resolution Process

The process should clarify roles within issue resolution in order to effectively manage intake, response and tracking in an efficient manner. Actions should include:

1. Build a process map for information and issue tracking within the organization.
2. Ensure the process map identifies who manages the information at what point and within established timeframes. If answers or responses aren't made during the assigned timeframe, the process map should allow for a reminder and/or sending the issue higher up in the department for resolution.
3. Make issue resolution the responsibility of each operational business unit. Far be it from Marketing or Business Development to "tell" operations or clinical departments how to resolve their service delivery issues. Most successful programs implement operational performance accountability and issue resolution systems with the support of the CEO,

COO and VP of Quality or Medical Affairs.

4. Have each department or service line identify a go-to person accountable for researching and responding to the physician regarding the issues as presented. This person may work with others, but is primarily accountable for the issue and response.

5. Provide the physician representative with a few criteria in which to capture the issue (three to five key questions) to return to the operational "go to" staff for their resolution and response to the physician.

6. Make sure you have Senior Leadership's support in positioning Operation's need to handle issues.

7. Track the process in a database. Many of our clients use Microsoft Outlook or Access, e-mail, or their current patient satisfaction systems to manage the tracking, reporting and internal communication needs of issue resolution.

8. Pre-design messages for the physician relations representative to use when a physician presents a problem. For example, when a complaint is made, the representative's response could be: "Dr. Smith, I can appreciate your concern regarding operating room scheduling. While the reason or solution certainly is beyond my expertise, I know the VP of Nursing would be very interested in hearing your concerns and connecting with you. In order to provide her with some specifics, shall I speak with you or your nurse?" Then, "I'll provide the details I learn from Mary directly to Sharon Jones, the VP of Nursing. You should hear directly from Sharon in the next three days. I'll also keep tabs on this request and work to keep you up to date. But do expect to hear from Sharon."

The essence of the message is, "We value input from our physicians and have a process so that departments are able to be responsive to your concerns." The role of the representative is to convey that, while they're not personally responsible for fixing problems, they can clarify the issue and facilitate communication.

Managing and Sharing Information

For many organizations, the new physician relations program—like other new ventures—falls into the category of The Golden Child. There's lots of intrigue and interest surrounding the program, including grand hopes for outcomes. For some, this also includes a lot of curiosity in learning what others are saying about your program. As a program leader, you have a great deal of responsibility for managing this sensitive area.

As the manager of the program, build policies for the dissemination of information captured from physician interactions. Think through the appropriate channels for market intelligence, peer-to-peer, Leadership-only and complaints.

Physician opinions—whether about people or programs—need to be carefully framed, shared and managed without overreacting. Too often, organizations fall victim to comments. One physician may raise an issue and suddenly the entire leadership team is in a frenzy trying to fix it. They're better off taking the time to explore if there's a general consensus on the issue; what the options for resolution might be; how long the problem has been occurring, and so on; and then asking one member of the leadership team to design a recommendation.

It's a classic case of too many cooks spoiling the broth. The obvious outcome is that the internal team also becomes numb when there are several crises in a week—each one demanding personal attention.

Review your internal plans for information management and make sure to:

- Clearly define a confidentiality and information sharing policy for the physician relations program. It's easier to expand the reach of information-sharing as needed, rather than retract information that was shared too broadly.
- Communicate issues according to the issue resolution process, track, and trend and make sure there is senior level accountability for implementation of the process.
- Communicate trends in the monthly report, with cumulative reporting of percentages on a yearly basis. For example, "86 percent of surgeons targeted for retention indicate there is difficulty in scheduling cases with less than one-week lead time in our operating room."
- Communicate physician-to-physician issues related to any clinical competency, ethics or physician-directed concerns directly to the VP of Medical Staff (and, when appropriate, to the CEO). For discretion, these issues or concerns typically aren't logged into the common database.
- Communicate service opportunities directly to the COO and service-line leadership. Document within the issue resolution and/or client management database for tracking purposes.

Physician Relations Management

While the chapters on structure and staffing talk about the reporting relationships and types of positions for this strategy, it is important to clarify the role of the individual providing leadership and management for the physician relations effort.

In some cases, someone in the management team has experience with physician relations. If it's with the relationship sales model, then that staff member may best be suited to initiate and run the program. However, in most organizations, this experience isn't available, so it's important not to house this program under someone who sees physician relations as problem-solving or event planning. It won't yield the desired results or satisfy Leadership in terms of results.

Usually, the physician relations program reports to a Senior/Vice President/Director level. This person needs to have regular access and communication with Leadership and be able to serve as the internal champion and buffer for the representative. Large healthcare organizations sometimes add a Director of Physician Relations or Referral Development position for the day-to-day management of a large field sales force.

While a staff member serving in this role may also have other assigned duties such as business development, marketing and physician recruitment, here are some key management accountabilities for a person overseeing physician relations:

- Executing system-wide sales and marketing responsibilities of developed services to identified target customers.
- Developing physician relations infrastructure and sales integration internally and organizational efforts to develop referral relationships with physicians, their staff and other identified referral sources.
- Demonstrating organizational and key strategic service line results as determined through strategic, business and sales planning process.
- Appropriately staffing functions and supporting initiatives through performance management and compensation systems.
- Providing staff with training and development to ensure appropriate relationship sales skills and internal product knowledge.

- Managing system integration and coordination of all service-line sales activities at facilities. This includes the portfolio of services packaged for each identified target market. Activities include sales call coordination, customer profiling, promotional materials and presentation of service offerings.
- Implementing and managing system-wide standardized sales tracking and reporting software and protocol for all product lines at facilities.

Six Key Attributes for an Effective Physician Relations Manager

---

1. Ability to work strategically at the leadership level and tactically at the physician representative level
2. Respect from operational colleagues and the medical staff
3. Ability to use data and planning tools to build an effective physician relations business and sales plan
4. Ability to communicate internally and externally
5. Commitment and passion for the strategy
6. An added plus: previous experience in the field selling to customer populations, especially physicians

---

The Administrative Duties of the Manager

For the manager who has direct oversight for the physician relations function, here is a list of core administrative duties to get you started:

- Program business strategy and sales planning
- Research to support program rationale, budget and structure
- Budget

- Position control management
- Position descriptions
- Performance standards
- Compensation plans and payout formulas
- Recruitment process and tools (in conjunction with Human Resources)
- Orientation
- Training

Some Thoughts on Orientation and Training

Orientation:

While many programs assume the current hospital orientation will serve a new hire in this position, the physician relations manager needs to think about the additional orientation a staff member might need to be successful in this position. The orientation may include core components that all representatives are taught; other components can be customized to meet the specific needs of the representative.

For example, if the manager has recruited someone from outside the hospital, the new representative may need special instruction in medical terminology, exposure to the organization's culture, key clinical services, and internal introductions to all Leadership, key specialties and specialists prior to going out in the field.

We encourage all physician relations managers to build a 90- to 120-day orientation and training plan that includes exposure internally and externally, meetings with key services—as well as a debriefing and field observation to determine the representative's skills level and gained knowledge.

Here are some important components to include in your orientation:

- Introduction to all key service-line leaders and "go-to" experts for services
- Introduction to key leadership and medical staff
- Hospital operations, processes and protocols as they relate to physician relations and core services
- Review of current "physician issues" with discussion about standard hospital messages and responses
- Review of current issue resolution process and key staff involved
- If the new staff member doesn't have a clinical background, provide medical terminology and quick review of clinical offerings

- If the new member doesn't have a sales/marketing background, provide relationship sales training, field and phone training and sales management process review

Training:

Beyond a basic orientation plan, many physician relations programs invest in classroom training for their representatives and sometimes include service-line leadership. While there are lots of standard sales training programs available, you need to select one that's customized to healthcare, physician relations and, if possible, to your organization's needs. You'll want a training program that provides core skills, scripting,

models and scenarios of relationship selling with physicians and one that provides in-depth exposure to sales planning, prospecting and client management.

"We have a 90-day orientation process for our new liaisons. The salespeople are chomping at the bit to get in the field. It pays off in the long run to make sure they have done their homework and they're ready. This is important for both their internal and external credibility. One of the keys to orientation is making sure the salesperson has an overall understanding of the organization. Even if they're going out to sell one product line, they need to be prepared to answer questions about any part of the system. Healthcare is very complex: Your liaisons, even if they're not going to know everything, have to be connected to resources and have a good organizational understanding. We have our liaisons shadow in just about every clinical area of the hospital before we let them loose. That gives them product knowledge and also gives them connections and internal relationships."

Donna Teach
Vice President, Marketing and Public Relations
Columbus Children's Hospital
Columbus, OH

In addition to these basic training elements, a manager also should provide:

- Field observation and staff development

- Skill review and training with interactive role-play in regular staff meetings
- Message and script development as needed
- Annual conference and/or internal training sessions for professional development
- Training and development recommendations as a part of their annual review and performance evaluations
- Database or computer training to support tracking and reporting needs of program

Here are some topics a leader can include in the ongoing training repertoire:

- Staff evaluation and development
- Field observation and management
- Travel and expense management
- Internal communication plans
- Message development and utilization
- Sales planning in assigned territory
- Tracking, measuring and reporting systems and staff training
- Product knowledge and integration into strategy
- Tactics and messages to progress the physician referral relationships

The Strategic Role of the Physician Relations Manager

Because the manager is often the individual responsible for the implementation of the physician relations program, part of their job is strategic oversight of the process. The manager must have a clear understanding of the Board's and Leadership's expectations of the program and, to a certain extent, provide those two groups with a look at what's possible/feasible based on firsthand field knowledge.

The manager is responsible for implementing the business plan—a document that's been created from your insight. This is the person in the process who can sit on both sides of the fence, being the one to say, "I know you're interested in having us promote neurology, but our field intelligence indicates that there's a three-month wait to get a patient in for an initial work-up."

The manager also can help balance how much effort is placed on retention vs. new business strategies and must be the person who consistently manages role expectations. It's an important point: For so many organizations, the role starts clean with the representative doing face-to-face visits. But, over a period of time (and quite innocently), the representative is asked to take on more and more jobs "since they're out there anyway." The manager's job is to ensure that the people in the field—specifically hired to develop relationships and enhance referrals—are allowed to successfully develop physician referrals.

A note for mature programs on the management process:

Continually evaluate the current program and its results and design mechanisms for your program's innovation, growth and ongoing staff development. This is a challenge even when the program is working well, but don't become complacent. Stay on top of physician's needs and expectations of your organization, service-line innovations, marketplace competition and staff's need to stay "fresh" in their messages and positioning with physicians.

While this chapter isn't all-inclusive, we've tried to provide insights and direction for key management issues that have arisen in our years of doing these jobs and in assisting clients in their personal program implementation. The issues you and others in your position encounter will continue to evolve as programs mature and healthcare organizations push physician relations programs to the next level.

The role of the manager of this function requires multi-tasking and the ability to live in both the strategic and tactical worlds required of physician relations. In most cases, business development and marketing leadership lend themselves to these positions well because they're already involved in service-line marketing, integration, strategic and business planning and customer communications and marketing.

If you come from the clinical arena and physician relations is a new assignment, you can find success by networking with other physician relations managers and/or gaining an internal marketing ally. Don't be afraid to enlist others' skills and experience in your quest for an effective team!

Tips to Take Away

For those just starting out:

1. Ensure Leadership's buy-in at the strategic level. You can't grow these programs from the ground up and expect success. They have to be built and communicated from the top down in terms of a leadership-endorsed strategy.
2. Build an internal communications plan for ongoing messages and reports about the physician relations program.

3. Develop an issue/service resolution process, tracking and reporting system. Have Operations or Leadership manage and own accountability for this process and communication to physicians as to results.
4. Clearly define the administrative and strategic duties of the physician relations manager/director or vice president. Identify key characteristics and competencies required to be successful in this position, fit the organizational culture and ensure adequate program start up and ongoing management.
5. Build a plan for growing the organizational structure and infrastructure. Plan for success and how to grow your current staff as well as additional staffing or support needs.

For those growing or reorganizing their structure:

1. Review the leadership commitment to the physician relations strategy. If it's lagging or has changed since the program started, create a method to revisit the strategy with Senior Leadership and re-engage a leadership sponsor for your program.
2. Interview some of your key internal customers to learn their perceptions of the physician relations program and needs in terms of communication about service opportunities, issues or product development needs. Develop an enhanced internal communication plan to integrate suggestions and recommendations for increased tracking or reporting methodologies.
3. Review the issue resolution process and reporting tools. Capture input from the physician representatives and some select referring physicians about the issue resolution process, responsiveness and key areas for improvement. Again, work with the internal team accountable for issue resolution, develop system or process enhancements.
4. In most cases, managers at this level do well with the strategic duties and overall organizational support in terms of business development

and marketing. But field management and ongoing skill training of the physician representative can fall by the wayside. Revisit your position accountabilities, review the time allocated to the physician relations program and staff, and fine-tune your field and hands on support of their efforts. Most importantly, get in the field with your team.

5. Review the strategic and business plans that impact upon physician strategy and relations. Identify ways to advance the program in terms of growth, retention, loyalty and satisfaction of physicians. Ensure your team is properly positioned to support key operational and programmatic areas that are in development with plans for launching or engaging the physician as a key customer. You want to make sure you're a critical part of that process, not an afterthought!

Chapter 7

Evaluating Your Program's Performance & Effectiveness

"I know not any thing more pleasant, or more instructive, than to compare experience with expectation, or to register from time to time the difference between idea and reality. It is by this kind of observation that we grow daily less liable to be disappointed."

Samuel Johnson, 18th century English writer

At the leadership team's weekly meeting, the VP of Marketing says, "XYZ Clinic's recent physician survey indicated that too many of their own staff had little idea about all our organization offers. I'd like the opportunity to create a physician relations function so we could use face-to-face visits to communicate this. I'm sure we'll get referrals from it."

The CEO replies, "We had one of those and it ended up costing money with no returns. I don't think that is the solution. If you think we can get business as a result, show me the proof."

At this hospital, "proof" was just another way of saying, "Show me you can produce new business and then I'll support additional development of the program." While the CEO didn't much care about all the specifics, if he could see a shift in referral volumes as the result of a program, he was the first on board with the approach.

The VP of Marketing knew what she had to do: She'd work with the planner to evaluate the data and look for some targeted areas to grow referral business. After showing the CEO her intentions, she was hopeful he'd give her a little time to get the program on its feet so they could do it right and get some early results.

Back in the old days, hospitals often initiated physician relations programs simply because it was "the right thing to do." More often than not, the programs established today are created to meet specific and measurable goals for the organization. The basic economics of healthcare are such that only programs that prove value can be considered. There's a lot to celebrate when it comes to a sales-based referral development program—in particular, the reward of clear and measurable outcomes. But that's assuming you define what you'll measure and have the ability to track business into your facilities.

Beyond the organization's push for outcomes, evaluating your progress gives you a reason to pat yourself on the back and celebrate your success—and it serves as a taskmaster to help you look at your program, warts and all, and discover what needs to be tweaked or completely overhauled.

At its core, the evaluation process allows you to see:

- If the program is focused on what the organization needs
- If the program is executing per the business plan and other plan components

- If the representatives are doing what they were hired to do
- If the program is organized efficiently and effectively to deliver desired results
- Where there are opportunities learned through the evaluation process that can help you continue to grow

In this chapter, we'll show you how to build a tracking and evaluation system that takes into account both quantitative and qualitative factors. We'll also discuss why it's important to examine your process in several areas of your organization.

Defining the Criteria for Measuring and Evaluating Your Success

To be most effective, evaluation should be a multi-layered process that involves examining several different levels. It's not enough to simply look at one or two areas to judge your success. You need to take a comprehensive view of the activities and results generated from your physician relations efforts.

Many organizations make the mistake of expecting the physician relations effort to be all things for all people. The result, of course, is that the program implementers generally end up doing only a fair job across the board. Bottom line: They're never really able to give any areas enough focus or attention to gain the measurable results that the organization is waiting for.

The CEOs we work with consistently give four key reasons for wanting a physician relations program:

- To grow physician referral business
- To increase or maintain physician retention
- To enhance physician satisfaction and/or loyalty
- To stem existing referral business leakage

To achieve those goals, the program's leadership must clearly define up front *what* they'll evaluate to determine the program's overall success. From there, your leadership team can assign a percentage of time to be spent in each of the other areas.

For example, if the program is focused on new business development, the representative may spend 60 percent of their time in the field working with physicians who split their business or currently use other facilities. In the remaining field time, they may visit the current loyal physicians to ensure satisfaction and prevent leakage.

While this sounds logical, many programs put the heaviest emphasis on visits to their existing staff—with little or no effort on the heavy splitters or non-admitters. This approach doesn't allow much time to go after new business. The message here: Make sure the approach matches the expectations. And clarify it on the front end.

There's no cookie-cutter method for creating an evaluation process. But your program evaluation is pre-determined by the processes you've put in place thus far—from the business plan to performance measures to staff management. Obviously, then, your evaluation for some areas will be quantitative and, for others, qualitative. The essence of all good evaluation is the ability to track what's learned, to take anecdotal stories and/or data or trends and use them together to paint a picture of what you have and what you need. And it all starts with the ability to track.

Developing a Tracking Program

To successfully track outcomes, several elements need to come together within the organization. Obviously, Leadership will be looking for cause-and-effect links—a questioning process that sounds like, "What generates the new business and how much business comes as a result?"

Leadership many times wants to only track and measure the result, not activity to get the result. The reality is that sometimes the referral cycle (result) is long. And because we know that the representative has to engage in activity to effect change, we believe there's a need to measure the activity level of the representative.

Clearly then, there are two elements within the tracking process:

1. Looking at the activity responsible for creating the business; and
2. Looking at the actual business generated.

Life would be easier for everyone if this could be done in one fell swoop but, more often than not, it takes two separate tracking mechanisms to complete the process.

The first component is the responsibility of the physician relations team. Based on the sales plan, the manager tracks the representative's activity, detailing the activities in place that create the relationship and opportunity to earn/retain physician business. The most effective tracking, generally done in a sales management software program (we'll discuss that later in the chapter), delineates a tightly defined process for each visit.

To properly track the representative's activities aligned with targeted physicians, you'll need to have physician profiles entered into the database. Most hospitals have pieces and parts of physician profiles housed in a variety of areas and based on the needs of that department. Most of the profiles are only on those physicians who are admitters, so profiles may need to be built for those physicians who are outside the current medical staff but seem likely targets for referral development opportunities.

Mining the Physician Information

The starting point for any tracking, then, is to create physician profiles that provide their background. Beyond the usual name, specialty, age and practice partner detail, you'll want to know practice/business details: how they're currently referring—culled by evaluating the trended data from the business plan. Work to identify where they may be underutilizing you.

While early on, this is as much intuitive as data driven, you have the opportunity to look at referrals across service lines and determine if there are referral gaps. For example, if Dr. Smith seems to send patients to every specialty area except oncology, this is worth noting and working to understand in your face-to-face dialogue. So is the intuitive situation where Dr. Jones, a young family physician, used to send a large number of cardiac patients to you. But the number of cases for last year is less than a quarter of the volume it was before. Use the information to move ahead with your plan and targeted questions.

Tracking Pertinent Encounters

Central to the function (and to the long-term success of your program) is tracking the number of face-to-face visits with physicians. This details who was seen, the purpose of the visit, what occurred during the visit and the subsequent actions. We strongly recommend that you create categories within drop-down menus in the database, as this information needs to be defined and quantified.

Beyond the face-to face visit, you can follow other activities integral to advancing the relationship. These may include:

- Visits and meetings with office staff
- CME attendance to introduce a physician
- Bringing specialists to a primary care physician's office
- Getting a regional physician to attend grand rounds
- Meeting new physicians at a social event

The representative and their supervisory team can evaluate who's being seen and break that down into the actual percentage being seen to retain existing business and the percentage visited to get new business. Using the statistics, the manager may see where a representative is getting "stuck" in the selling cycle or if a person is using only one tactic or activity in their effort to progress the relationship.

A key step in gaining new referral business is connecting the referring physician with your medical staff expert. The representative is responsible for understanding what areas the referring physician or their group is interested in, then facilitating a discussion or presentation from your specialist. *These meetings, too, need to be tracked.* Again, the recommended approach is to track specifics so that details can be quantified, such as specialty, number who attended and the actions the representative will take after the presentation to determine interest and referral opportunity.

Keeping Office Staff in the Loop

Office staff is a critical hub in the wheel. And while the relationship with the physician is primary, there is a need for the representative to develop credibility with the internal team as well. Many times, in the consulting role, we've been told, "In our community, the office staff decides where those referrals are sent. I think they're the primary target."

Yes, this is true—until a physician walks out of an exam room and says, "I've had it with ABC Hospital. I don't want anything further to go there." At that moment, no relationship you have with the office manager will overcome this referral hurdle.

The lesson? Nurture a primary relationship with the physician and support it through a relationship with the office manager. Today's representative needs to be the physician's liaison for solution and referral details. Manage the role and the office hierarchy appropriately to assure your program owns that role.

As you track visits with the office staff, reference these conversations as you move forward in the implementation process. The representative will detail who was seen in the office, the messages or materials provided and the intelligence learned—all to identify further opportunities.

Accessing the Data

Many organizations struggle with deciding who should have access to the representative's tracking data and logged notes. There may be a desire to have many people involved—but there's a lot of very specific detail that needs to be managed and understood in the context of the relationship.

Generally, the sales management database is the responsibility of the supervisor of that program. If the CEO is actively involved on the relationship side and wants access, obviously this is someone to accommodate. Otherwise, there should be a central contact for internal people to call, generally a secretary who's responsible for overall data base management and who can be available to share details on an as-needed basis.

Everyone with access to the data must understand the rules of confidentiality. Put a policy in place that says the data can only be used after a discussion with the physician relations team. There are times when a tidbit of information, taken out of context, can destroy the credibility of the representative. Those situations often start simply because someone is anxious to get the scoop or be the first to respond. But, regardless, they set a dangerous pattern; too often, physicians will catch on and quit talking!

Data Input and Integrity

The representative needs to have field tools that allow for ease of entry and eliminate the need for duplication of notes. Most representatives use a laptop with their sales tracking software. Bad data entry habits can develop if the representatives are not required to do regular input and synchronize with the central database. Our recommendation: Have the representative take brief notes with the physician and input the details into the laptop after the visit or, at a minimum, at the end of each field day.

Ensuring data integrity is a battle for many departments. In physician relations programs, there are some recommended ways to keep data clean and viable:

1. As we discussed, have Leadership mandate the tracking expectations with time lines, type of tracking to be done.
2. Have a central coordinator, generally an administrative assistant or the department's database support person, assist with keeping the central database up to date. This includes detailing what will be entered, formats and creation of drop-down menus and support with the reporting functions.
3. Train the physician representatives on how to use the system and to maintain data correctly to benefit their reporting to Leadership.

To create a cause-and-effect referral chain, identify the primary care physician and then the specialist. While organizations do an excellent job of detailing the admitting physician and which specialists are treating these patients, often there are gaps in showing who generated the initial referral. Because that person is generally the target for the physician relations representative, the system must commit to capturing this detail *when the patients are admitted.*

Reporting

In any industry, people are fond of saying, "If it isn't documented, it wasn't done." In healthcare, we put a little different twist on it: "If it wasn't documented in a way we can find and interpret it, it doesn't count."

Such is the saga of many of physician relations programs. Intuitively, you feel like you're making progress; yet, there are so many fragmented reports that you can't see the forest for the trees. The most successful programs have cleared a path and are continuously looking for succinct ways to detail what the program has accomplished within a report.

Types of reports for consideration:

Most successful programs use several levels of reporting. The first and most obvious—a monthly activity report completed by the representative to detail what was done. If the program has sales management software and the software to support report writing, the bulk of this detail is fairly easy to produce. This report is a key tool for program management as it details who was seen, actions toward progressing the relationship and generally offers good insights and market intelligence.

If your organization wants to communicate the general activity and intelligence to others internally, the management team is often charged with creating a monthly team report. If you're in this position, work to provide a high-level, one-page report for the senior leadership team that shows what was accomplished, the impact and the intelligence.

Referral reports for Leadership:

Within healthcare, numbers sell. Look at the program's impact every quarter according to its goals—referral development, retention and/or satisfaction and loyalty. Is your organization plagued by ongoing internal operational challenges, but your program has a percentage focus on retention? Then call out the key issues presented by physicians—again, not through personal stories, but by the percentage of time that certain issues were mentioned.

For example: In the first quarter, Jolene the representative made 180 physician visits. Of those visits, 40 were to surgeons. Eighty-two percent of the surgeons she visited said they would use Acme's outpatient surgery suites more often if they could get time on the schedule.

Present the quarterly program and issue report to the CEO, COO, CFO, and VP of Medical Affairs, in addition to the department that immediately oversees the program. You'll want to prepare and distribute this report consistently; use the same format, day of the month, look and style. Doing so inherently speaks to the focus and consistency of the program.

One or two times a year, in the management updates, offer a presentation on fieldwork outcomes and findings. This is your chance to give a verbal accounting of the program and its contribution to the organization's goals, and re-affirm the organization's internal commitment to the program.

Creating quality reporting for Leadership is so logical. Yet, in the haste to get the reports out and the nature of finding the time, they're often put together without the attention to detail they deserve. The most effective remedy is to create a template, assign a due date, enlist Information Technology's support in getting hospital-based data to meet the due date, and then schedule a period of uninterrupted time to complete the report.

"I presented our results data to the service-line operations and also shared it with the Chief Communications Officer. He saw this and said, 'I want you to bring this to Senior Leadership.' So I did a similar sort of presentation. When I was finished explaining what the program is, how we're measuring results and what kind of results we're seeing, the CEO's comment was, 'Why don't you have 12 of these people?'

You couldn't ask for a better endorsement than that. Having that sort of support is invaluable, but you can't get it by just saying, 'We think it's good.' Doctors in my physician-led organization say, 'Show me the details.' They want the data. Until I had the data, I don't think I would have gotten that same sort of response."

Kathy Dean
Associate Vice President, Marketing
Geisinger Health System
Danville, PA

When you've completed the report, read it through and ask yourself these questions:

1. When I read this, will I know what the physician relations representative accomplished in the last quarter?
2. Will I clearly understand the program's goals and efforts to meet those goals?
3. Will I know where we have internal vulnerabilities according to the physicians?
4. Will I gain the "outsider's" pulse on the market by reading the market intelligence in the report?
5. Will I be able to articulate what this program is doing for the organization moving forward?

Organizational Goals Drive Tracking and Measurement

Based on the goals of your program, you'll likely want to evaluate the impact of the program through referral patterns. Unless your program is purely in business to improve satisfaction of the existing physician referral base, you'll need to rely on the hospital database to determine the referral/retention impact. With that in mind, how do you go about "getting credit" for getting and keeping business for the organization?

Evaluating the Business Impact

Through experience, we've learned that there are fundamentals that—if put in place at the start-up—will enhance the organization's measurement capabilities. While logical, the steps in the process are often skipped because all the interest and attention is placed on "just getting out there."

1. Determine what you can measure. Based on the business plan, trends and targets, there's a sense of what needs to be measured and what's in place to make this happen. Some facilities admit that they're presently incapable of doing a good job of tracking the original referral source.
2. Make sure what you can measure has a direct correlation to your program goals. If the program is asked to grow business, the measurement yardstick must be able to show a cause-and-effect relationship.
3. Evaluate accepted measurements for the organization. Step back and make sure that what you're proposing to measure provides a perceived value for the senior leadership team. For example, if you suggest measuring calls to the physician referral line, but Leadership sees that service as a glorified answering service, you're not likely to receive the respect for the effort that you'd hoped.
4. Decide who gets credit for what on the front end. Ugly, bitter battles ensue internally when several departments try to claim the same new business in their ROI reports. This happens when Marketing says the new business was because of the ad they placed in the state family practice journal, the clinician says it was because of the new technology on the unit, and the physician relations representative claims it was because of their targeted visits. Note that if several new ROI-based programs are being initiated, there may be a split credit. That's fine—just make sure to decide up front.

5. Stay consistent. Once you have something in place, resist the temptation to improve, enhance and change it each quarter. Even if the first attempt wasn't the best, keep the process in place so that you have something to trend and look at over a period of time.

"Through One Call, a centralized communication system, we have the technical capability of measuring the timeliness of our hospital staff responses to requests for telephone consultations from community physicians. We can also measure the amount of time it takes for our hospital staff to reach the busy physicians in the community. Those data have served to reinforce the fact that beyond a few outliers, the timeliness of telephonic communications to and from this hospital is generally good. In addition, these computerized reports have assisted us in making decisions with regard to staffing One Call and also allowed us to test market certain approaches to expedite connections between physicians."

James Shira, MD
Medical Director of Physician Relations
The Children's Hospital
Denver, CO

Quantitative Analysis

A quantitative analysis is often challenging because of past tracking methods and because of the challenges with "who gets credit" for growth internally. Work though the internal processes first, then determine which approach will work best for you.

Whether your organization needs retention or new business development, you'll need to match where the business is coming from and understand why. More specifically, you'll need to find out what referral was from what practice, and the result of your program's targeted physician relations efforts.

Model 1: Physician-Specific Measurement

In a perfect world, the organization could see the number of new referrals to specialist offices, the number of new patients using outpatient services, and the number of patients admitted for inpatient services—and then be able to clearly show the new referral pattern was because of the physician relations representative. Truth is, it just doesn't happen that way.

As we discussed, there's often a lack of good data on the primary care physician who initiated the referral. Organizations do an excellent job of tracking the specialist or hospitalist who admitted the patient. But you'll rarely find an Admissions area that takes the extra effort to ask, "Which doctor do you see in Saltville for colds, flu and your general health needs?"

The result: Organizations often have fragmented information about who initiated the referral process. If a program really wants to do it right, it seems worthwhile to invest in getting this detail started so there is a path for recognizing where the business really comes from.

We define this model of measurement, used by many organizations with excellent success, as the *Physician-Specific Measurement*. Here's how it works:

Quarterly, the representative will detail the physicians he's targeted. This generally includes all the key-targeted physicians seen in the last three months. This list will then be "matched" against the inpatient and outpatient data (if you're lucky enough to have this in good shape as well).

The type and number of patients and revenue is detailed and the representative is "credited" with creating that referral relationships. As these programs shift to more retention, the same method applies. In evaluation, however, you'll use trended data and look at the baseline, rather than crediting the representative for all the business.

Model 2: Service-Specific Measurement

A seasoned representative is always focused and prepared to discuss any and all services of interest to the physician, including the organization's key strategic services. Organizations that want to grow in two or three service lines need to provide the representative with messages about the service lines the organization wants to promote.

However, because this is a generalist model, based on the physician's interest, there will be times when referrals are generated to service lines that aren't the key strategic lines. While measurement in this model only includes the key services, there's some spillover into other services that also contribute to the organization's overall success.

To put this model in place, the organization needs to look at past trended data. Ideally, that's three years' worth, in order to determine growth in the service line. Now's an excellent time to assess if there are "other factors" like payer, changes in physician staff, and/or competitive threats that have or will dramatically impact the service.

From there, you'll need to make decisions about what growth to expect without the program and then come to an agreement that any growth over X amount (again, measured quarterly) will be credited to the physician relations effort. Generally, there are just two or three key areas that are evaluated. While it's not as tightly defined as the physician-specific model, change is evident and measurable in the service-specific model. And it's the one most organizations use today.

Model 3: Organizational Growth

The third model used by organizations looks at growth in total for *all* service lines. Organizations who use this model generally have a number of representatives in the field charged with promoting the full continuum of services.

The organization looks at trended growth across all service lines and then says, "We've grown at X percent each of the past three years." But it also takes into consideration why and if there are other market influences projected to change this in the course of the next year.

The result is that there's agreement that growth would be at X percentage without the program and anything over that amount will be credited to the physician relations effort. Something to note, however: This program does come under tremendous scrutiny if there aren't detailed conversations about "who gets credit," as we discussed earlier.

Which Should You Use?

If your program is totally focused on retention, your best bet is still the physician-specific measure. In the event that won't work, likely because of the current data capture, you may use the organizational growth model. Or, if you're only focusing retention on a couple of services, the service-specific model will work as well. The tough part with a retention focus is proving the physician relations effort was the reason there was no loss of business. This really requires clear negotiation about how the program will be given credit. As we discussed, this needs to happen on the front end of the measurement agreement.

For that reason, you may have a compelling need to add satisfaction and potential revenue outcomes data to the mix—that's if you know the relationship efforts have resulted in more profitable procedures coming your way or a shift to a more profitable payer mix as a result of the representative's efforts.

How Much Growth Should You Expect?

It's the hardest question of all for the outsider. The best expertise for determining market opportunity comes from within the organization. Using the internal data and good market intelligence, you have an opportunity to estimate where growth opportunity exists and how much of it you can expect to capture.

The other key component in framing market potential is the input gained by the representative in the first two visits. After meeting with the prospective referral source, the representative should have a good understanding of where there's an opportunity to shift business and by how much.

Three pieces of information are combined to develop a forecast for the program: 1) internal data on current use and potential, internal intelligence about the physician and practice; 2) field representative intelligence and; 3) level of opportunity and openness to shift their referral.

Because we know that changing major referral patterns is a 12- to 18-month process, many programs look for small shifts or changes in outpatient volume and increased business from splitters to detail potential earnings for Year One. New programs can certainly be a budget neutral expenditure—even in the first year, if there's a focus on new business development.

Qualitative Analysis

Beyond the numbers, many organizations use programs to enhance satisfaction, create better relationships and trust, and shift loyalties. While very difficult to capture in a quantifiable way, you do need to demonstrate the qualitative benefits provided.

For many organizations, whether they're facing capacity restraint or adequate numbers of specialists—or if they're a dominant player and simply need to maintain—the focus is much more on the qualitative side of the relationship. These programs need to stay in contact with key physicians; often, the goal is communication and making sure physicians understand that the hospital values their business.

Some organizations continue to strive for more loyalty and commitment from their active medical staff. They use the representative to sell the medical staff on using more services, getting more involved with Leadership or other members of the medical staff.

We doubt the loyalty of the past can be replicated for our current generation, but good communication can go a long way in creating a more harmonious working relationship.

Some hospitals that actively solicit input from the medical staff via a physician satisfaction tool are very concerned about negative opinions and attitudes of the staff. Subsequently, they implement the physician relations effort with the goal of increasing physician satisfaction.

Again, communication is often at the center of many of the physician's complaints. If the representative is to be successful with this endeavor, there needs to be a hospital-wide endeavor to ensure internal commitment and help the physician feel the effort is honest and credible. The representative is then charged with finding more ways to offer value, bring back information on the physician's needs and expectations and create mechanisms for connecting people who are on the leadership with the physician and his staff.

If your program's goal is to enhance satisfaction, you need an organization-wide effort to effect change. Once the organization has made strides toward enhancing satisfaction in a specific area, then the representative can communicate this information to the physicians and encourage them to "try again." Good follow-up will be critical to both ensure it met their expectations and, assuming it did, to assure them of their wisdom in reporting the past issue and being willing to try a new approach.

Growing the Program, Beyond the Dollars

The most successful programs know they need to continue to cultivate relationships with physicians to grow the business—but they also know there's much more to the physician representative's job. This person needs to consistently look for ways to add value to the relationship, to assure the referral sources their input is valuable and to look for ways to better work with the internal audiences.

An aspect of adding value (one that's often overlooked) is working to keep the program vital and fresh from the inside out. Seasoned representatives know it's easy to become complacent and, from time to time, a bit bored with the routine.

Managers can help stir the pot and motivate representatives by helping them create personal innovation challenges, look for new ways to engage physicians, try new communication approaches, learning about new services and understand more about the current offerings.

Long-term success and program growth requires continuity in the representative's role—and that takes a commitment to keep the role and the internal enthusiasm for it visible.

Successful programs are very aware of their organizational impact. Furthermore, others within their organization can clearly articulate what the program does and how it serves the strategic needs of the organization. Getting to that point however, is no easy matter. The process of deciding how to evaluate shouldn't be an afterthought. From the onset, as data is gathered, tracking programs are developed, strategies are created, there is always that clarity of goal about what the expectations are to be.

As programs shift to stronger quantification of outcomes, there is a compelling need to communicate the impact to the key leadership. It's the job of physician relations to clarify what they will deliver in qualitative and quantitative terms and then demonstrate those results in consistent and concise reporting.

"Using a physician relations strategy has given us the most valuable information you can imagine. The physician relations program allows us to keep our finger on the pulse and be alerted rather quickly when our docs are unhappy about an issue. Another valuable asset is the ability to quantify anecdotal information so that we can effect change. Without the database to track issues and comments, information was more or less hearsay. Now we have reports that demonstrate on a quantifiable basis the percentage or number of physicians who are dissatisfied about a particular issue."

Gail Callandrillo
Vice President, Planning & Market Research
The Valley Hospital
Ridgewood, NJ

Tips to Take Away

For those just starting out:

1. Take the time to establish a baseline for measuring the program's success. Don't merely "get out there" and assume you'll be rewarded.
2. Clearly define how you will track the field activities and the referral results. Work with Information Technology, Finance and/or Planning and Leadership in the program development phase.

3. Establish what you're going to track and measure, then stick with it. Constantly changing measurement criteria and methods will leave you second-guessing your impact.
4. If you have limited field intelligence, it's difficult to do an accurate forecast. Do a good job of budgeting for expenses, then use the first three months to gather field intelligence. Use this insight with the numbers to complete a more accurate forecast.
5. Develop an internal reporting model that's consistent and meaningful for the person who receives it. As with all things, if they can't understand it, they won't buy it.

For those growing or reorganizing their structure:

1. Evaluate what worked in your tracking and measurement strategy. Keep those things and re-tool the rest.
2. Conduct an informal audit of the internal stakeholders who have received past reports. Find out what they felt was helpful and if there were one thing they'd like to see, what would it be. Don't promise you'll give them everything they want, but do compile and look for opportunities to enhance the internal reporting process.
3. Rely on data and your intuition to create forecasts of referral development growth within your region.
4. Take time to evaluate the staff and their professional growth needs. Explore ways to give them support with ongoing skill development and role-growth.
5. Make sure you focus on the number-one need for the organization; then match your return-on-investment tracking to that need.

Chapter 8

Incorporating Sales Planning in Your Program

"Few people have any 'next,' they live from hand to mouth without a plan, and are always at the end of their line."

Ralph Waldo Emerson, essayist and poet

Acme Hospital had decided to formalize their physician relations approach by staffing a fulltime position. They had completed a pro forma, identifying revenue and volume levels to justify the cost.

Jane, the new representative, had previous experience in the hospital's home health program. She was well respected by physicians and their office staffs and was knowledgeable about the hospital's services. One year into the program, Jane presented a report to her CEO. While strides had been made in retaining key referral patterns and physician satisfaction, little had occurred to grow new referral relationships locally or in surrounding communities. Acme's CEO wasn't dissatisfied, but she asked Jane to focus her next year's program efforts on delivering results that matched the organization's strategic plan.

Jane had never been asked to do this—and was challenged to craft an approach that would help her deliver on this request. After talking with other contacts, Jane knew she needed a sales plan to help her identify who to target for this and how to stay on course. Using the strategic and business plans for the hospital, Jane developed a plan that identified key sales and marketing objectives with quantifiable results forecasted and for each called out key strategies and tactics that would ensure she was successful. The sales plan created an organizational focus for physician relations as well as a personal road map for Jane to follow and report on throughout the upcoming year.

Sales planning is a crucial process and tool for all organizations that plan to use, or already use, a face-to-face staff to focus on retention and growth. It's the mechanism for translating the hospital's goals into sales objectives that are measurable and defining the strategies, tactics, resources, timeline and forecasted outcomes for each objective.

There are two types of sales plans:

1. A team plan—designed to support the overall physician-related strategic initiatives.
2. An individual plan—designed to define the individual sales representative's territory or pool of physicians.

Organizations with more than one physician relations representative will use both types of plans. In this case, the team plan will serve as a roll-up of the overall physician relations planned activities to achieve objectives. It also will identify resource requirements to support the planned activities that may include marketing communications, collateral materials, hardware/software, etc.

Good sales plans, whether team-based or individual, are derived from the organization's overall strategic plan, key service line's business and marketing plans. They should reflect Leadership's strategic initiatives while communicating how desired outcomes would become a reality.

Sales planning is the representative's tactical action plan that serves as the roadmap to accomplish their goals and objectives. The individual plan confirms for Management that the representative clearly understands their mission and has strategically thought through how to deliver. For the physician representative, the sales plan must identify the specific strategies and tactics they'll use to get the desired relationship sales results.

Beyond helping the representative to their ultimate success, sales plans can:

- Help you be efficient and effective
- Keep you organized, on schedule and focused on the right activities
- Enhance physician follow-up, communication and depth to the relationship
- Identify barriers to success and present solutions for a successful sales approach
- Track your results against planned goals
- Help identify other department's support required to successfully market and deliver on the promise to physicians

A sales plan is dynamic; it's not designed to sit on a shelf. The plan should be an actively used road map, updated every 90 days to revise activities, forecasted results and/or shift in strategies based upon organizational direction.

In this chapter, we'll take you through the steps of creating a plan, provide some samples to build on in your program and show you how to integrate some of the things you've learned in the previous chapters to move the process along.

Why Have a Sales Plan?

- Sales plans translate the overall goals of an organization into personal sales and marketing activities focused on a targeted population with specific forecasted results. This provides the sales staff with specific quantifiable activities they must do in order to successfully deliver the desired outcomes.

- Sales plans also serve as a means to confirm Leadership's expectations of the physician representative role in the field and what will be measured or defined as success. This also sets up an internal platform to educate Leadership and peers about what the physician representative will be accountable for and what their role is focused on.

- Creating a sales plan is the business development and representative's opportunity to communicate the activities and results that can be directly attributed to their positions.

The Sales Plan Pay-Off

While sales planning is sometimes thought of as a tedious and painful process (especially the first time around), it becomes the critical glue to properly setting the stage for the physician representative's success.

A strong sales plan also helps your organization to:

- Build internal clarity as to roles and responsibilities
- Develop a clear articulation of agreed-upon goals and desired results
- Have a strong ability to manage accountabilities and staff performance
- Develop more efficient territory management
- Focus on targeted prospects and service lines
- Create a proactive, strategic approach to the marketplace
- Gain the ability to report value and outcomes

What Do You Want?

To ensure the success of the plan and its results, identify the number-one desired result for the representative's territory. For example, if your goal is to grow the business, it should be reflected in:

- Who the targeted physicians are
- What the frequency and depth of face-to-face meetings are
- The planned actions for gaining referral commitment and timeline

---

Starting the Planning Process

The sales planning process should begin with Management setting overall relationship sales goals and objectives for the representatives. If there isn't a "sales" manager for this function, it usually will be facilitated by Business Development or Marketing, with input from Administration.

Management should ensure the development of the sales plan either through providing a framework of objectives and/or a template or model of the desired sales plan. Management may need to assist the representatives to think in terms of what tactics and what frequency will deliver the desired results.

Once the overall goals and objectives are established, each representative needs to review their territory and assigned pool of physicians to determine how they'll contribute. Measurable objectives need to be set (combining performance standards and strategic goals) for each representative reflecting the market opportunities within their assigned territory.

Key steps for the physician representative in plan development:

1. Review organizational goals and determine how your personal efforts will support achievement.
2. Review and assess all services to be offered to make sure they meet the identified physician's needs and will achieve the desired referral volume outcomes.
3. Assess the competition in terms of your goals, their approach and how you will differentiate your approach, messages and offerings to succeed.
4. Build tactics and activities that will keep you focused on achieving the desired results with the appropriate targeted physicians. Build into the plan the frequency of visits, phone calls and follow-up for efficient and consistent management of new and current referring physicians.
5. Build a mechanism to track your results against your plan. Be prepared to analyze and fine-tune quarterly and at year-end.

To stay current, your sales plan should be updated quarterly. And while some organizations make their sales plan an annual task, we've found a 90-day, action-oriented focus helps the representative stay on top of critical tactics and focused on measurable results. What's more, the quarterly plan aids in keeping the content brief. Its quantifiable actions and results focus allows the representative the ability to fine-tune their approach based on what's happening in the marketplace and on previous results.

A Sample Sales Plan

A solid sales plan clearly delineates your organization's goals and identifies measurable objectives that match the desired outcome. For each objective, you may have several tactics to support the actions.

For example, here's a slice of the Acme Hospital plan with the goals and some of its objectives, strategies and tactics:

Goal:
To generate new referrals into the organization, especially for cardiovascular and the ambulatory surgery center.

Objectives:
1. Increase cardiology referrals from "A" physicians by 4 percent in 2004.
2. Generate new referrals into ambulatory surgery center, averaging 12 surgical procedures scheduled per month.

Strategies:

Strategies are the approach you'll use to fulfill your objective. Acme Hospital may choose to conduct needs analysis updates on all "A" physicians in order to match their needs with your solutions. Their strategy includes:

1. Conducting qualitative and quantitative market research in your area to identify your customer base
2. Reviewing data and fine-tune targeted physicians by current referral patterns, geographic location and desired DRG/populations
3. Identifying current referral "A" physicians that aren't optimizing organization for cardiology and conduct educational/needs analysis meeting to determine ability to ask for their referrals into service line
4. Identifying non-referring "A" physicians and focus on a 90-day window to get appointments
5. Reviewing current physician profiles and market intelligence to build "door-opener" and key messages to gain referrals

Tactics:

Tactics are the methods you will use in the actual implementation of the strategy. They may include (but aren't limited to):

1. Building a targeted segmented prospect list according to predetermined criteria
2. Developing a "sales" work plan and timeline to map out your phone calls, face-to-face appointments and follow-up—day-by-day, week-by-week, etc.
3. Developing and managing a customer profile to solidify your baseline of information

4. Identification of additional activities and offerings to use with targeted physicians to progress the relationship
5. Mapping out the frequency and geographic management of targeted "A" physicians for optimum results, focusing on shifts in outpatient and ambulatory and long-term inpatient referrals

Sample Sales and Marketing Action Plan

Objective	Increase referrals by 4 percent for Cardiology
Strategy #1	Meeting with targeted physicians
Tactics/Activities for Strategy #1	Identify for each tactic/activity your planned start and end date, who is responsible and measurable outcomes for this tactic/activity.

	a. Develop list of targeted physicians
	b. Analyze priority to Cardiology
	c. Code A, B, C for Cardiology
	d. Call 12 offices per week for appointments
	(Remember, you'll also have some appointments with surgeons to discuss ambulatory to get to that 15 to 18 appointment per week average)
	e. Convert 8 per week into appointments
	f. Conduct 8 face-to-face meetings with MDs
	g. Convert first meeting to second meeting
	    a. Specialist site visit
	    b. CME
	    c. Office staff tour
	    d. Repeat face-to-face visit

Strategy #2	Marketing Communications
Tactics/Activities for Strategy #2	Identify for each tactic/activity your planned start and end date, who is responsible and measurable outcomes for this tactic/activity
	a. Develop letter from Chief about Cardiology b. Send 20 letters per week to list c. Code list for Cardiology update fax d. Develop outcome flier for Cardiology e. Learn current CME offerings for Cardiology f. Promote CME g. Provide physician representatives with marketing information on CME for promotion to their lists

When Your Plan is Done—What's Next?

Now, the sales manager or Management should:

- Ensure that each representative's plan properly supports the organizational strategies and service lines.
- Make sure the plan is focused on the targeted physicians for each strategy and that the representative is using the appropriate approach in terms of efficiency and consistency to achieve results.

- Use the sales plan as a 90-day action plan with each representative reviewing their own targets, focus, planned activities and forecasted results.
- Use the sales plan to communicate the approach and outcomes to Leadership.
- Centralize events and marketing communications efforts with assignments to the appropriate departments. This ensures that the representatives aren't distracted from their primary focus of developing relationships with assigned physicians.

Reading the Crystal Ball

You may notice that, throughout this chapter, we talk in terms of desired results and/or outcomes. One of the reasons relationship sales fits so well with growth and customer strategies in healthcare is because it's measurable and can report on outcomes deemed valuable to the organization.

This requires a fine balance of realistic expectations of relationship sales and the length of time to produce results. Management and staff need to understand that referral patterns do not change easily or lightly. Nationally, outpatient referrals may shift in as little as three months. Inpatient referrals (which are much more physician-to-physician-based and may be deeply rooted in long-term relationships) may take anywhere from 9 to 24 months.

So, we recommend outcomes be framed in realistic timeframes and be balanced with additional measurables that define the depth of the changing relationship. Other sample achievables may include:

- Letter and/or invitation
- Opening phone call
- Opening meeting and relationship information (Attended X number of CMEs or hospital educational events)
- X number of meetings conducted or coordinated
- Needs analysis meetings (Thoracic surgery referrals driven by pulmonologist presented)
- Interim solutions and/or issue resolution as interim step to potential referral
- Customized responses to needs via activities to progress the referral relationship and access to organization
  - Specialist presentation
  - CME
  - Tours
  - Office staff support and/or access
  - Outreach clinics
  - Exposure to equipment or new service
  - Grand rounds
- Deeper, more progressive conversations that the referring physician to a commitment

In order to frame realistic outcomes, Management and the representative should use organizational and service-line data trended over three years, if possible. Beyond the data, Management and the representative should review the market nuances, political environment, and capacity/access issues and apply the "reality snapshot" to the data and outcomes.

"Develop a strategy, then remember to follow it. Also, we think the outreach committee model for educating and networking with physicians has been a success. It is comprised of physicians and management from each service line or program who are available to meet with physicians and practices in the communities to educate and present their available services, answer questions and understand their needs. Their involvement with the practices has greatly reinforced our commitment to the physicians, their staff and their patients."

Betsy Hayden
Director of Corporate Health Marketing
Carolinas HealthCare System
Charlotte, NC

Get Real

Make sure you use a dose of reality in sales planning and forecasting reasonable activity volumes and outcomes. For example, if you have a pool of 1,500 physicians, one representative and a 28-county area, it becomes important to manage the reality of a 40-hour workweek, drive time and access to physicians. Be practical. You'll need to either target your pool more closely or you'll need more representatives.

Integration of Performance Measures Into Sales Planning

If you happen to have started the book at this chapter and haven't already developed performance measures and evaluation tools, we recommend you visit Chapters 4 and 7. Once they're designed and approved, these tools and measures should be integrated into the representative's personal sales plan. The planned quantity of activities and results should be reflected within their sales plan while identifying their plans and timelines for achievement.

Sales Reporting: Planned Versus Actual

An important requirement for any physician relations program is the ability to provide reports to internal customers. As we've discussed throughout the book, outcomes are critical to the long-term success of this program and Management should ensure that Leadership and key service lines receive updated reports on what the program has accomplished for them. This report should meet three goals: It should be customized for each to reflect the key information points they value; it should be done monthly for key leadership team members and quarterly for service-line leaders; and it should be one page, bulleted and easy to read.

Key categories for sales report information include:

- New Business
- Pending Opportunities
- Market Intelligence
- Upcoming Events
- Issues (quantify and prioritize)

"I can't underscore enough that effective sales planning will move market share. You can build volume through a well-executed formalized physician sales approach. How many other things do we do out there—how many ads do we run, how many direct mail campaigns do we do—but there's always that question of value on the other end: We spent the money, did we really build the business? There's a body of proof with the formalized sales approach that, if appropriately executed and tied back to your strategic plan, it will grow your business. From my vantage point, out of the tools in the tool chest, this is a pretty exciting one."

Wayne Sensor
CEO
CHRISTUS Schumpert Health System
Shreveport, LA

(Editor's note: In mid-2004, Sensor assumed the CEO post for Alegent Health in Omaha, NE.)

Sales Automation: Tracking, Measuring and Reporting—A Manager's "Must Have"

A critical "must-have" is tracking implementation of the plan. Sales automation programs give teams the ability to track, measure, report and communicate about the physician, market intelligence and the program's outcomes. Many organizations will optimize the systems they already have in place, while others will utilize an "off-the-shelf" sales contact management system that's customizable for the physician relations program.

Programs such as ACT!®, GoldMine® and SalesLogix® are available online and/or at computer software stores. Regardless of which one your organization ends up using, the software will need to be customized to reflect the activities, results, sales plan targets, performance expectations and other internal measurements such as service lines represented, issues, etc. Reports generated by the automated system can incorporate all sales planning, performance standards and detail actual performance and results against the plan.

Sales Contact Management Software Resources

Act!: 480-368-3700; www.act.com

GoldMine: 800-776-7889; www.frontrange.com/goldmine/

SalesLogix: 800-643-6400; www.saleslogix.com

Sales Force: 800-667-6389; www.salesforce.com

Sample Document: Sales Planning Worksheet

Since sales planning is the right thing to do, but skipped by many organizations in their zeal to get out into the marketplace, we've provided a checklist and process to assist Management and the representative in the development of their sales plans. Remember, there's no right or wrong way. It's just important to do it—and in a way that works for you and your organization.

Starting Point

1. Define the representative's assigned territory, including geographic and pool of assigned potential and current referring physicians.
2. Create definitions for the A, B, and C categories of physicians.
3. With Leadership and staff input, assign A, B, C coding to physicians.
4. Determine visit frequency for each category.
5. Determine objectives and desired outcomes for each representative's territory.
6. Review desired outcomes and total pool for referral development. Identify activities and personal sales focus for daily/weekly efforts to deliver outcomes.
7. Discuss issues such as politics, leakage, growth and opportunity to shift market share.
8. Review marketing communication support and events.
9. Determine how results will be tracked, measured and reported.
10. Review strengths, weaknesses, threats and opportunities (SWOT) on your own program and the competition.

Sales Plan – Key Points

1. Territory Analysis – Should include physician populations, estimate of potential, need for program/service, leakage issues, current referrals by program/service, potential referral—sources by program/service and/or location, and competitive information.
2. Tactical Plan to Achieve Results – Should include activities that are direct sales, events, marketing and service with key

stakeholders generating referrals. Activities might include: face-to-face appointments with physicians, practice managers, office and business managers, hospital leaders (rural executive staff) for outreach referrals, CMEs, events, service line or facility tours, and/or presentations.

3. Steps to move the physician toward more referrals – Build action-oriented steps that a physician can engage in and that you can track to demonstrate their referral patterns and engagement with your organization.

   Sample steps:
   a. Returning to the physician's office with service-specific information or a clinical specialist to present the update
   b. Engaging the physician in a short-term project to share insights and recommendations to the hospital about a specific issue
   c. Setting up a physician-to-physician meeting
   d. Getting the referring physician to attend a CME, grand rounds or participate in a teleconference or presentation at your hospital

4. Identify the number of physicians (potential or current referral source) to be covered, the frequency of visits, number and type of visits (new, follow-up, service, physician versus office staff, educational), travel time and time per visit (estimated). Make sure to focus on time spent on prospecting, retention, growth and service.

5. Identify market intelligence and client information to be captured and kept up to date by the salesperson.

6. Detail the methods in place to track, measure and report on results of sales and marketing efforts.

1. Prioritize products and services to meet potential and current referral sources' needs and your organization's desired outcomes.
2. Develop positioning statements – "What's in it for me?" (WIIFM) in terms of benefits to your referring physicians to do business with you, your organization and program.
3. Create dialogue-oriented questions to interact productively with prospects and clients.
4. Write scripts to position products and services appropriately matching client indicated needs.
5. Train staff on products and services, packaging, promotion and access.
6. Prepare staff to manage issue resolution, delivery and capacity issues and operational coordination.

Tips to Take Away

For those just starting out:

1. Don't worry about format. There's no right or wrong way to write a sales plan. Develop one that you can use and that Leadership will easily read. Consider using software so that you can import lists of targeted physicians per strategy and monitor results against plan.
2. Be consistent in creating, updating, evaluating and enhancing the plan. Review the strategic plan annually, work on reviewing data from past year's efforts and organizational desired outcomes. Identify where sales can provide results and how.
3. Build in accountability steps such as who is the responsible party for completing a task. Some sales tactics may involve other departments or internal staff and their follow-up is critical to the relationship

management process. Calling out accountabilities helps inform and engage all staff in successfully building referral relationships.

4. Realize that Management needs to show interest in the plan and mentor their team in working the plan. Use this as your means to communicate at all levels in the organization as to approach, focus, required resources from other departments and what outcomes will be credited/measured as a result of this effort.

5. Don't let the plan become the outcome. It's not a thesis. It should be user friendly and succinct.

For those enhancing or reorganizing their plan:

1. If you haven't done a plan in the past, add this to your program enhancement using it as an internal education and confirmation tool.

2. If possible integrate this into your budget planning process to evaluate past performance, provide recommendations for program growth and enhancements (such as added staff, new markets or services and/or enhanced results.) Use this as a service-line forecasting/planning tool to coordinate sales targets and results and craft mutually agreed-upon expectations.

3. Provide physician representatives with a template sales planning tool. Conduct a workshop on sales planning and have them craft their 90-day plans for your personal review. Encourage them to focus on activities they can directly be accountable for that will deliver the optimum results to the program.

4. For other activities such as events, marketing communications, etc., collect those into an overall physician relations sales plan for coordination with appropriate departments in terms of budgeting, timing, results and staff support.

5. Use sales planning as a means to enhance staff focus and performance. Review sales plans quarterly for each representative and evaluate them in the field (observe calls and debrief). At year-end, review their results versus planned.

Chapter 9

Advancing Physician Relations

"Now, here, it takes all the running you can do to keep in the same place. If you want to get somewhere else, you must run at least twice as fast as that!"

Lewis Carroll, author, from *Alice In Wonderland*

Acme's physician relations program is continuing with little fanfare or glamour. The representatives appear to be in a rut and Leadership pays less attention to the referral volume shifts than they did when the program was just starting out.

At the last leadership retreat, the CFO said, "I'm not sure we need to continue to allocate resources for two people in that program since it seems we've stabilized our referral business. With limited new business, this is an expensive allocation."

As the VP of Business Development, you hear the message loud and clear: It's time to re-energize the program. You know that only the

programs with positive drive can sustain themselves at Acme—and you
know the value in your physician relations program.

In healthcare today, there's little room for complacency within any
program, including physician relations. Money's tight and labor costs and
workforce challenges are at the forefront. What's more, reimbursement is
a constant challenge for many organizations. It means business
development initiatives must add and demonstrate value or they'll be
subject to cuts or elimination in many markets. Physician relations
programs are faced with that feeling of, "We need to do something
different here," for three primary reasons:

1. The model and expectations don't match.
2. The program is stagnant.
3. The market has changed—there's more competition, physicians are
   leaving, and new specialties are popping up.

To sustain long-term customer relationships, the physician relations
program has to have something new and fresh that keeps the internal
and external teams interested and engaged.

Programs that are stagnant or threatened may be in that position for a
couple of reasons. First, it could be the kind of program that's been fixing
problems for a long time—and while there's recognition that they need
the program to focus on business growth, to date it just hasn't happened.
In all honesty, that's generally because there's no one to take over the
problems or because the person in charge of the program is more
comfortable in the role of service than sales.

Problem solving is a nice thing to do. But if the organization is interested
in shifting to growth and new business development, then the program
will need to shift to that level of accountability. It's only the rare

organization that's willing to fund costly programs because they're "the right thing to do."

Historically, many hospitals had enough financial cushion to hire liaisons to trouble-shoot for the medical staff. While some of those still exist, more and more hospitals have launched a concerted effort to put outcomes with expenditures. These programs are looking to continue to use people in the field, but place more emphasis on new business opportunities.

The second reason a long-standing program may be stagnant or threatened: plain and simple, they're in a rut. They've been successful in growing the business, but as the prospects turn into customers it is harder and harder to generate new business. All the first-round business has been captured and, basically, the team's getting a bit bored and the organization assumes the referrals would have come in anyway.

In this environment, there's a tremendous need to innovate and look to new opportunities. That may include expansion of the targeted areas, going deeper within the existing referral base, or collaborating with others to open new product/service offerings or offer them in a different way. Keeping a pulse on the strategic direction of the organization will keep the program in step with the needs and expectations of the physician relations market.

This chapter will discuss how to analyze your physician relations program as it stands now—and how you can improve and grow your program to meet the changing needs of your organization and your targeted physicians (and fix the things that haven't panned out as you'd hoped). Take the time to reflect on your successes and failures, then ask the tough questions that can make your program even better.

Conducting an internal assessment of where you are and where you need to be is the best way to determine if the time is right for a mere tweak or a total program overhaul:

- *Take a minute and ask, "What have we learned?"* That includes the marketplace, your customers, your internal ability to deliver what they expect, the vision of your leadership team and the processes required to implement a sales function within a basically non-sales-oriented environment. This assessment is critically important to deciding where you need to adapt, how and why.

- *Use data, perceptions and intuition to determine what's working and what's not.* Look at how much labor you have and what the impact has been in tangible terms as well as the altruistic evaluation of doing the right thing.

- *Evaluate future strategies and their integration with the current goals of the program.* Make it a priority to evolve the program to stay in step with the future needs.

- *Review the strategy and desired outcomes.* Match staff's accountabilities and results to the plan. Ask the following questions:

  - Do you have the right staff focused on the right results in a dedicated manner?
  - Do we still have disconnects?

- Did you build an issue resolution process that looks great on paper, but in reality the representative continues to "fix" problems rather than handing them off to the designated operations person for management?

- *Determine the program's fit with current marketplace interest.* Beyond what the organization wants, what do the customers want and, in many cases, expect. Are these expectations in line with the priorities of your program? If not, can they be? If they can't, better re-think the internal piece. There's little value in telling the prospective physician they're wrong in their expectations.

- *Use the same process to determine which service lines are generating the most interest in the market.* If the organization wants you to push cardiology and all the regional physicians seem intent on hearing more about your oncology services, there needs to be a change in your approach and focus.

- *Assess where you've taken the physicians within a relationship continuum.* Do they trust, confide, and turn to the representative as a trusted source of information? Have each liaison rank their current relationships in their targeted market. While subjective, this exercise lets you know where you are and if there's a need for more training to move the relationship forward. Assess what the liaisons believe they're actively doing to advance the relationship.

- *Look at what's currently in place to differentiate the physician visit from other vendors or liaisons.* Challenge your thinking: "What can we do to enhance the value of the visit and differentiate ourselves from the competition?"

- *Evaluate the integration process to date.* Are there other internal areas or staff to be integrated into the physician relations strategy? Part of this process may be to look at how well Sales and Operations are working together.

Internal Assessment Checklist

Is your organization in good shape to move forward? Take these steps to find out:

1. Look at the original goals of the program.
2. Review the organization's overall business strategy.
3. Make a list of ways a physician relations program could affect key initiatives moving forward.
4. Assess the fundamentals of implementation.
5. Go back to the list. Refill the funnel.
6. Revisit your approach for keeping the leadership and other internal stakeholders informed.
7. Try something different. Look for new ways to advance the relationships and go back to the sizzle factor. This will keep the interest alive far beyond the vendor or tell-and-sell models.

Business Planning for the Next Phase

With the assessment completed, it's time to develop the business plan and create the strategy for where the program needs to go. If you've been planning with regularity, the numbers and trends will be easier to assess. Many times, it's easy to pull up an old template and just update the plan. That's okay for routine updates, but if it's been several years, why not try working from a clean slate in the areas of market intelligence, market opportunities and trends?

We're accustomed to looking at our organizations from the inside out. But remember that we may look very different from the physician's point of view. If you haven't done a SWOT (strength, weakness, opportunity, threat analysis) from the perspective of the referring physician in a while, take the time to do that exercise with Senior Leadership. In addition, list the program accomplishments to date—or, if you have an older program, in the last five years.

The elements of the plan, then, are consistent with what we defined in Chapter 2:

1. *Using the strategic plan, frame the marketplace.*
   a. Look at targeted physicians.
   b. Define expectations. List a percentage of time in each activity. For example, Retention 50%, New Business 30%, New Physician Mentoring 10%, Management 10%. This does change with a more mature program.
   c. Identify service lines that are candidates for a direct sales approach.
   d. Consider your targeting options. In some markets, the state database allows the team to clearly understand where all the business is going.
      i. Organizations are able to look at payer mix, who's splitting their business and by how much, and how market percentages are shifting by physician and by hospital.
      ii. Armed with this data, some organizations employ a splitter or targeted payer strategies.
      iii. These programs still offer service in keeping with all legal standards; they simply choose to use and

target this expensive marketing resource to the practices with the most referral potential.

    iv. Programs that can track to this level of detail enjoy tighter targeting and more measurable outcomes—and have their leadership teams interested in using a niche target approach.

2. *Acknowledge success to date and why.*

    a. Look at trended data and do a full analysis of market opportunities.

    b. Add a market intelligence portion to this analysis. Are there areas you're unable to break into because of political hot spots?

For example: Have you had good methods of learning early about loyal physicians in the region who are considering an early retirement? Or were you able to respond quickly when you learned of vulnerabilities with the competitor's programs? How did you get the details and how can you get more?

3. *Keep what's working.*

    a. Based on your assessment, you'll be able to determine which approaches are working best.

    b. Look at the details. Do you get more referrals from areas that have outreach clinics? Do calls to the access center increase after you do office staff receptions? Look at each of the strategies you've tried. If you can attribute good growth to them, include them in the next level of planning.

    c. If you're not able to show growth with a targeted practice, don't include it in the plan unless you have a strong rationale for testing one more time. (This is key in terms of time management and sales focus. Use the plan to re-target and remove the dead-weight tactics.)

4. *Consider innovative, trial ideas with a rationale.*
    a. Refuse to assume there's only one way to advance the referral development process.
    b. Try new approaches. Use education, print materials, phone calls, and/ or public relations tools to create something new to test.

5. *Continue to validate the leader's wisdom.*
    a. Within the business plan, spell out how you expect the physician relations program to be measured.
    b. Detail the plans for tracking and reporting
    c. If the physician targets remain fairly consistent, then forecast growth opportunities for the marketplace. You can use numbers of referrals or revenue and volume. It's best to break this down into the two top specialty areas you intend to grow and then detail how you expect to reach the forecasted dollars.
    d. Within the forecast, keep retention and customer service separate.

Who Has the Time?

Taking a program to the next level is not without its challenges. Often, while there are a couple of key members of a leadership team who are driving the interest, the masses are probably thinking, or sometimes saying, " Are you nuts? I'm barely keeping it together as it is. We have no time, no budget and actually no desire to offer to do anything more than we already have."

It's probably true—they're not sitting around looking for something to do! What the visionary team members need to help position is that if we don't change, innovate or add depth, the program will no longer have value. Change may require that we let go of some of the old patterns to create new ones.

Success requires that you add depth to what you can do and to the messages you provide. As you begin to advance the approach, work to gain involvement of others. At times, physician relations programs do fall victim to the very silo behavior that they so despise when working through some of the service-line thinking. It's not a job where you can be independently successful. Success depends on a team approach, so give up some of the control and trust that others in the organization are competent as well.

Obligations for Growth

Assuming your program is doing well, you've made small tweaks where necessary, and there's a lot of internal interest in more market growth, you need broad-based internal support to take the program to the next level. Within the organization, each group has its own obligations for growth.

Leadership

The ongoing involvement of Leadership is key to the success of any physician relations program. Often, you'll be faced with changes in the people and/or the structure, or the key members are now totally distracted with a new project. Pay attention and continue to assure the leaders of their wisdom in supporting this program. There must be a champion at the Leadership table, someone who "gets it" if the program is going to thrive.

In most organizations, you'll find outstanding systems of measurement for many things, but not for physician relations activities. Advancing the program generally requires knowing what you want to measure and how. To take it to the next level requires baseline data on the current market by physician. To get your hands on the data, or the ability to "drill down" to get the right data, may require Leadership assistance or intervention.

The final must-have from the leadership team is a clear focus on strategic expectations. Have a vision of where the program needs to fit in with the overall strategic plan and where the physician relations program can assist in making it happen. Leadership can help you set the course for the program to be a long-term approach to doing business with the right customers.

Program Leaders

The program leader has to have credibility with Senior Leadership to make sure ideas are heard, and outcomes generated by the team, receive their due. It's Leadership's job to paint a picture of the next steps when a new approach is being taken and the waters ahead are uncharted. Salespeople aren't always easy to manage and it's human nature to fall back to the old "we always did it this way . . . " mindset. The leader of the program needs to be attentive to the teams' adjustment to the advanced model during this period in order to set some clearly defined expectations.

The program leader will also be the one who can best recognize the need for additional training and development of the physician relations team. If the model is going to change, there has to be some relationship sales training for the representative and, in some cases, the internal service-line team. If tracking and targeting is going to change, there needs to be good internal support from the technical support and planning staff. Anticipation of training needs and the ongoing development and mentoring will be a big part of advancing the relationship.

Representatives

Any time you change someone's job responsibilities, it's a strain. Even for the representative who's bored to tears with his existing job, he can still have apprehension when the word's out about a new approach and new accountabilities.

Success in this role requires lots of tenacity and an ability to innovate. It also requires a certain level of playing by the rules and trying to do the job in the way Leadership intended—in good faith. It requires a willingness to re-learn, to re-think old habits and to put yourself out there in order to personally grow to the new level.

During times of transition, it's easy to want to take sides against the internal team, against each other and against even the physicians you need relationships with. Resist the urge to take sides. Give yourself 90-days with the new plan before judging. Take on the mental responsibility to understand that no one's trying to have you *not* succeed.

Advancing Internal Relationships

Beyond the need for better targeting and a physician relations program with more depth, there's also an opportunity here for better integration with other internal departments and services. Physician relations crosses all departments and services, so as the program develops there should be more rather than less emphasis on collaboration with other departments and services.

Use the list of targeted services to design an internal communication strategy for reaching out to these areas. Yes, it would be nice if someone else did the "reaching out" from time to time, but if it hasn't happened to this point, it probably won't—so just do it.

Internal marketing communication plans seem to work best when everyone understands their role and the agenda. The program leader is in an ideal position to support this, but shouldn't be held solely accountable for all the internal communication. The representatives need involvement within the reality of their roles in the field.

"We have amassed a tremendous amount of data we were able to distill down to concise dashboard reports. These reports are shared with the executive staff, the medical staff leadership, and with Board-level committees. I think it is very helpful for them to not just guess at what doctors are thinking and saying, but to really know that meaningful data is backing up their assumptions. Previously, the only doctors that we heard from were the very vocal ones, or the ones who were active on hospital committees. Now we get to hear from the 'quiet ones' too! I believe that this aids in long-range planning and in goal setting."

Beverly Miller
Director, Physician Relations
The Valley Hospital
Ridgewood, NJ

If you've never done an internal communication plan before, start small to avoid being overwhelmed. You may decide on two departments that you want to work more closely with—one that benefits from your services and one that you need. For example, you need Planning, and Cardiology needs you to generate new referrals for the program. Engage your bosses' agreement in this plan and process; if their peers ask them about your meetings, they'll be prepared to respond.

Do your research and find out who your contact person is, then start with an e-mail message that states your purpose: "I'm involved in expanding our physician relations program to the eight-county region. I'd like to learn more about your department and how the planning data could help me focus on the right physicians for our services. I'll plan to call next week to set a time for us to meet."

Go to the meeting prepared to introduce yourself and your role, and to tell the contact that you think there may be some mutual benefit to understanding more about their area. Bring your questions. Then, after the meeting, make a monthly connection with the department representative—whether it's by sending an e-mail, stopping by or calling.

Continue the dialogue by telling the department person what you've learned that's relevant to their job, and ask for help or advice in positioning or in extracting data or whatever you need. Just like making a new ally—here, both parties win.

Experts say that success in sales requires three elements in equal parts:

1. Product knowledge
2. Understanding of how to package the product according to access, schedules and who's who in the specialty area
3. Selling skills

The new representative faces a deluge of information to absorb. Most feel an overwhelming need to learn the products and services, in enough depth so they're comfortable in talking with the physician. At the same time, they need to learn how to gain access, which specialists are the right ones for which specific types of patients, and what the support services might be—it's all part of how to package your organization's offerings.

If the representative has sold in the past, the emphasis is on converting those skills to this new environment and then testing how to prospect, ask questions and present the benefits of working with the organization and its specialists.

This approach works well for gaining access and starting a relationship. However, many representatives struggle with taking the next step and creating the personal skill set that allows them to advance the relationship with the physician. Patterns are set in the early visits; yet, as the representative does more visits, they want to have more dialogue and advance the relationship. How do they do it?

Sometimes it begins by starting back at square one and revisiting some of the basics of sales. Is the current approach truly dialogue-based or has it fallen into more of a "tell-and-sell" approach? The very nature of a physician's limited time means the representative often has a tendency to talk about products and services—rather than engaging the physician in dialogue. This may work for a while, but inevitably you'll come to that bump in the road where there's not enough "new stuff" to share to make it worth the physician's time.

If the representative finds this happening, it's time to step back, assess the program and the desired approach, assess the skills of the team and then get the right skills and approach aligned with the desired expectations.

For many organizations, this means more or different training. The training should involve the entire team and give an opportunity to think about the approach, decide what needs to occur, provide the tools to succeed and then lets the team practice in a comfortable environment.

Advancing the Relationship

Beyond adapting the skill set, the representative is often challenged to consider innovations for keeping the physician's interest. There are many right ways to get physicians involved. Take the time to brainstorm ideas within your organization. Here are some ideas to get you started:

- Conduct mini-task force meetings. Invite regional and local physicians to a meeting on a topic of interest. Hold two or three sessions with a tight agenda and outcomes that can be implemented.
- Expand the circle of influence. Engage Leadership in working with physicians beyond the current circle in special task forces, projects or hospital-physician programs.
- Provide educational seminars. Select topics that showcase what you offer that they may need, then follow up with subsequent sales calls.

- Hold special events in the doctors' lounge. Go beyond donuts on Doctors' Day and create impromptu ways to connect with announcements regarding social events, new technology and people.
- Build internal recognition programs. Recognize those who write articles, or participate in extra meetings even those who did something extra for the Foundation Gala. If it's done on an impromptu basis, it can be fun and not expected.
- Create a contest for nurses to vote for physicians in various categories—Rookie of the Year, Best Story Teller, Easiest to Find . . .
- Provide food at the hospital, rather than their offices.
- Recognize key office staff. Send a pizza to the office, without a visit, but just to say," We know you've had a busy week, so enjoy." Or, hold a special training program in an area they've asked for.

As you advance the relationship, look for ways to recognize physicians' interests and talents and personalize the approach. Give them recognition in their communities and position their value to your organization.

The best representative makes sure physician relationships are developed over time with mutual respect and trust as the cornerstones. With that in place, there are tremendous opportunities for project involvement as well as support with the educational needs and referral opportunities. The ideal role for the representative is to be seen as a valued resource for the referring physician.

As your physician relations program matures, the intensity of figuring out the role and expectations shifts. Roles are understood—and with them, more emphasis can be placed on collaborative working relationships. Along with this comes the need to understand other value-added services and what areas might be of interest.

Many organizations believe they need to give the physician something to get referrals—whether it's business support, management services, a joint venture opportunity, etc. In reality, the things you really want to give are a sense of trust and a relationship.

Learn about the physician desires. Instead of following past patterns of "build it and they will come," determine what you can offer, then get input from those prospective referring physicians who will use it. It's a logical next step, but too many organizations forget to take the time to ask the physician for their input. Some areas of interest may include:

- Practice marketing
- Practice management
- Joint venture opportunities
- Clinical leadership and education
- Recruitment
- Access to a physician-to-physician call center
- Involvement in consumer campaigns, public relations stories

While some of these can be done without charging, many of them do require the not-for-profit to charge the physicians at fair market value. As you query the physicians on their interest, make sure you also discuss their willingness to pay a reasonable rate.

In advancing the program, clarify who will be charged with implementing these value-added offerings. Use the representative to solicit their interest, but charge other internal experts with facilitating the actual implementation.

This will let the physician continue to see the representative as the primary resource for referral relationships and for connections to other experts within the organization. For organizations interested in taking on the value-added approach, consider a process map similar to one designed for issue resolution.

As part of this process, the representative learns about the support services and the people charged with their success. You'll find great opportunities for internal networking and sharing of ideas, market intelligence and general brainstorming on next steps based on what you have and what the physicians want.

Is it All Worth it?

Change can be a painful process. Even when you know it's the right thing to do, you may still want to focus on tangible outcomes to prove it was worth it. Every program will have its own victories: Many will say they benefit from better visits, more outcomes and more trust at the physician level. In addition, advanced programs are seeing more physician involvement and more internal willingness—for both physicians and departments—to get involved.

Not surprisingly, success always leaves Leadership wanting more. The leaders in your organization will continue to expect the program to perform and bring results (and can you blame them?). Make sure you continue to communicate the priorities and establish realistic expectations.

The bottom line: An advanced program provides more and better opportunities for success. With more involvement, a stage set for innovation, a true dialogue-based relationship and trust in place, your organization can be in the right position to continue to enhance relationships with the medical staff and create a win-win environment for all.

Alice in Wonderland really did say it well: To be effective in today's market, organizations must continue to innovate and analyze what they need for the future and be willing to live in a managed state of flux. Successful physician relations programs have the ability to be self-critical and continue to work to improve and enhance their level of relationship, referrals and value for the internal and external customer.

Tips to Take Away

---

1. Evaluate your current program and physician environment—both internally and externally. Take an objective look at whether you're meeting expectations. Try to look at your program and its organizational needs from the outside in.
2. Realign the strategic priorities with the market opportunities and update the plan. If you've had success in the program to date, take the current realities and craft a plan that allows you to grow to a new level.
3. Be willing to give up old approaches as you take on new accountabilities. Many, many physician relations representatives suffer from overload because they try to do all of the old jobs and take on ever-pressing new responsibilities.
4. Grow at a personal level in knowledge of the product and packaging and in personal skill set. Refuse to get in a rut and feel like you "know it all." Once you have the basic skill set, you'll be able to experiment with nuances in style and approach that push you to the next level of relationship success.
5. Initiate opportunities for integration and communication within the organization. There is an ongoing need to help the staff understand

the world from the outside perspective. They can't initiate this themselves, so take it on and welcome those opportunities for their interest and learning.

Special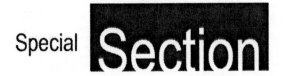

Words of Wisdom & Thoughts on Physician Relations

"Experience is not what happens to you; it is what you do with what happens to you."

Aldous Huxley, author

Many of you know the adage, "You can't be a prophet in your own land." We thought it might be helpful to share some of our client's insights that might either confirm the path you're taking or perhaps provide alternatives to your approach. It's been interesting to us to see trends in physician relations—these shifts and the subsequent debriefings with our clients have helped us develop many of the "must-haves for success" we've shared with you in this book.

This chapter is built from interviews conducted with clients from hospitals and health systems of all shapes, sizes and geography. It is a collection of e-mail, phone and editor interviews. Each client tells their story in their own way—and their candid answers show that there truly isn't one set process.

Their responses demonstrate that it takes structure, flexibility and hard work for an organization to determine what will work in its culture in order to achieve the desired outcomes for successful physician relationships. We hope these insights and anecdotes will help you as you build your own story on physician relations.

Todd Flickema
Director, Business Development
Avera McKenna Hospital & University Health System
Sioux Falls, SD

What have you gained by using a physician relations strategy?

Time is a precious resource for everyone. When this resource is in short supply, it makes establishing relationships that can bear the fruit of increased referrals that much harder. I think this is where devoted positions to business development have been critical to our success.

These people (business development/physician relations) are able to establish and nurture these relationships because it is their main task and not an addition to seeing patients (doctor) or running a department (hospital patient care director). With these relationships in place, they are more easily able to put on the table our growth areas and positively affect business for us.

Some of these representatives actually rise to the level of being seen as an asset to the practices they call on. They become our eyes, ears and messenger in the field. This is also an effective use of our internal customers. They can spend more time seeing and caring for patients and we bring them in for discussions with outside customers when the representatives have already laid much of the groundwork.

What measurable results can you report?

Across the board, we have seen increases in referrals. Some of this may be consistent with our growth in medical staff, but no doubt our efforts have moved up the natural timeline of gaining new referrals.

What would you do differently next time—in planning, execution or evaluation?

You need to have clear measurable goals for representatives and clear and consistent direction from senior management. You need constant feedback to your representatives both objectively and subjectively. They need validation that their efforts are making a difference and that they are executing the wishes of senior management. We did not always appreciate the extent to which they need this validation, but understand it now and our recent enhanced efforts here have been well received by the representatives.

What ongoing challenges do you face with your program?

Keeping the sales staff motivated and making sure that your incentive plan is competitive. You have to always reflect on these things, but at the same time don't change direction too often or else you risk sending confusing messages to your sales staff and disengaging them from the sales process.

Going forward, how do you intend to grow or reshape your program?

We strive to further quantify our needs for growth in order to set goals for the sales representatives. These goals have to be consistent with senior management and ongoing communication from senior management to the sales representatives on the goals helps keep their focus and validates their hard work.

.

Judy Blauwet
Senior Vice President, Business Development
Avera McKenna Hospital & University Health System
Sioux Falls, SD

What have you gained by using a physician relations strategy?

Success of an organization is about maintaining and growing market share. How to get there is simple in terms of knowing where to focus an organization's energy. It is all about building and maintaining positive relationships with and between physicians, especially primary care and specialists. Key elements include getting to know one another, listening to each other's needs and desires, and providing solutions. Mutual respect and trust become core to the process.

For Avera McKennan, the physician relations strategy proactively facilitates building the healthcare delivery process. Our representatives have built their own trusting relationships with regional physicians and hospitals, as well as with Avera McKennan physicians and mid-level providers. This allows them to get into offices/open doors/introduce new physicians and/or services that would never otherwise be possible. It also places them in a position of accountability, as the senior management of the organization has come to rely on them as valuable members of our healthcare team.

What measurable results can you report?

In the years prior to and including fiscal year 2003, Avera McKennan's growth in admissions was in the 3 percent range annually. In the first six months of fiscal year 2004, our growth in admissions was 5.6 percent.

What would you do differently next time—in planning, execution or evaluation?

In addition to what Todd Flickema offered in his comments, I would add that we have learned that in hiring, we need to focus on hiring for "sales." The core elements include tenacity, the ability to be told "no" and still feel good about themselves, quick thinking, as well as solid listening and communication skills. Taking time to hire the right person is worth the energy put forth in gold.

What ongoing challenges do you face with your program?

Our program has grown and matured to a point where it is now valued within the organization. But keeping a lid on ongoing operational expenses is always a challenge. I think the other challenge is finding good salespeople for healthcare—that can fit the internal culture and develop the business externally.

Going forward, how do you intend to grow or reshape your program?

We may make some changes in territory/role as we modify our strategic initiatives—e.g., more of a focus in the network vs. the primary service area, or more of a focus on corporate sales as opposed to physician relations in the network.

Pam Bilbrey
Senior Vice President, Corporate Development
Baptist Health Care
Pensacola, FL

What prompted the need in your organization for a physician relations strategy?

Certainly we want to continue to build loyalty among our physicians. I think one of the things that really prompted us to take it to the next level was, a couple of years ago, we divested ourselves of our employee physician strategy. We had at one point about 48 employed physicians—family practitioners and internists—and this group went out on their own. In our community, there're all open medical models and a lot of splitters, among at least two of the hospitals, if not three. Without an employed physician strategy, it became critical to continue to have open communication with our physicians and build relationships and loyalty to our healthcare system—and to learn how to provide better services to our doctors.

What have you gained by implementing this program?

It has helped us gain better insight into the physician perspective in the delivery of healthcare services in our community. It has provided us with actionable information regarding ways in which we can enhance the physician-hospital relationship and helps us identify unknown service recovery issues.

What measurable results can you report?

We do an annual physician satisfaction survey which indicates improvement. We conduct physician focus groups to ascertain how well we are doing in engaging physicians in organizational improvements. Results include few disruptive physician incidences, physician support of Baptist Health Care public policies.

What would you do differently next time—in planning, execution or evaluation?

We would start with some formalized training for those making calls on physicians and their offices and have a more structured approach and follow-up system in place.

What are some must-haves from your perspective, or advice for your peers?

An organization must have support from Senior Leadership and a commitment to make contact with physicians and involve physicians in the decision making process. It's important to involve physicians at all levels of the organization. A few ways Baptist Health Care engages physicians are:

- New physician welcome receptions held several times a year
- Physicians and their families are invited to an annual Doctors Day dinner and IMAX movie
- Having physicians serve on the board of directors
- Physician birthday list distributed to all department leaders
- Frequent thank-you notes to physicians for going beyond
- Ongoing leadership development sessions for physicians

What ongoing challenges do you face with your program?

How to keep the communication fresh and consistent and keeping physicians informed. Challenges also include dealing with physicians who only see the MD side of healthcare and requests from physicians to change/resolve an issue/situation that is inappropriate (this applies to only a few, rather than the majority of physicians).

Going forward, how do you intend to grow or reshape your program?

We will be looking for some physicians maintaining volume, others increasing volume. We'll set a percentage amount of decreased calls to our physician action line, a telephone number that physicians can pick up 24/7 and register a complaint about something. We'll also be looking for increased engagement of our physicians—more attendance at meetings, more participation in CME, more physician committee chairs at the hospital. Those sort of markers will be important for us to look at as we focus on bringing physicians into the planning and operations of healthcare.

Betsy Hayden
Director of Corporate Health Marketing
Carolinas HealthCare System
Charlotte, NC

What have you gained by using a physician relations strategy?

Having a simple, but well-refined strategy enabled us to focus our efforts on our mission—or desired outcome—more than would have occurred if we did not adhere to a strategy.

What measurable results can you report?

Our program began in 2002. In the first two quarters of 2003, we saw a steady increase in referrals in targeted service lines. More important and measurable are the number of physicians we have assisted in networking with other physicians (primary care physicians or specialists). This has increased physician perception of the liaison value to them.

What would you do differently next time—in planning, execution or evaluation?

For execution, we'd allot more time for continuous internal education, about the hospitals, programs and services. This has been extremely important.

What are some must-haves from your perspective, or advice for your peers?

Develop a strategy; then remember to follow it. Also, we think the outreach committee model for educating and networking with physicians has been a success. It is comprised of physicians and management from each service line or program who are available to meet with physicians and practices in the communities to educate and present their available services, answer questions and understand their needs. Their involvement with the practices has greatly reinforced our commitment to the physicians, their staff and their patients.

What ongoing challenges do you face with your program?

It's been a challenge to acquire all the referral information and data to determine current referral patterns.

Going forward, how do you intend to grow or reshape your program?

We have plans to grow the number of physician liaisons and expand their geographic areas, as well as to continue to involve more hospitals, services and programs in ways to add more value to area physicians.

James Shira, MD
Medical Director of Physician Relations
The Children's Hospital
Denver, CO

What has your hospital gained by using a physician relations strategy?

We have learned how to gather meaningful data regarding the dynamics of pediatric medicine within our community and region, and then synthesize the information into strategies that produce significant positive impacts on our hospital's relations with community physicians. Next, we have begun to generate, among referring pediatricians and the family practitioners, recognition of just how much we appreciate and value not only their referrals, but also their participation in hospital affairs.

The physician relations program has implemented systems that have measurably improved our two-way communication with referring physicians. Each day, we learn more about the expectations of referring physicians; at the same time, we have been successful in developing an understanding and sensitivity in the community concerning the many demands on hospital-based, university-associated academic physicians.

Christine M. Rhodes
Director, Physician Relations and One Call
The Children's Hospital
Denver, CO

What have you gained by using a physician relations strategy?

- The liaison program provides the visible face for The Children's Hospital in the referring physician community to demonstrate our commitment to working in partnership with them.

- We have gained an organized voice to referring physicians regarding services, customer service.

- We offer a vehicle to gather the opinion of the referring community and utilize it in hospital decision-making.

What measurable results can you report?

By integrating One Call with our physician relations program, we are able to control the quality and speed of service for physicians who enter our system through the call center. We have a goal of getting the urgent caller connected with the physician consultant they need in two minutes or less. Our call center software can track this and we are working towards a goal of 90 percent of calls connected in two minutes. In February 2004, we were at 87 percent.

We are getting closer to being able to have regularly at our fingertips referral information on the physicians we visit. This will allow us to track changes in referral patterns and attribute them to physician relations interventions.

What are some must-haves from your perspective, or advice for your peers?

- A reporting relationship that ties the physician relations program to quality and operations and support from the highest level of administration.

- An adequate budget to support what the department is being asked to do (we are fortunate to have this but I hear others don't).

- Decide if your physician relations program needs a global focus or a service-line focus.

- Evaluate what the competitors are doing in your market and make sure you are doing something of more value for the referring audience.

What ongoing challenges do you face with your program?

- Holding operational departments accountable for process improvements based on the feedback the physician relations program gets in the field.

- Holding faculty at a teaching hospital (who are not employed by the hospital) accountable for customer service related issues.

- Getting everyone who hears complaints, concerns (and compliments) to report it to a central repository (physician relations) so that information can be presented in the aggregate.

- Recruiting, training and retaining good staff.

Going forward, how do you intend to grow or reshape your program?

We are looking to add an internally focused physician relations representative who will be responsible for relationships with internal faculty and house staff and some retention. This individual will plan and implement orientation for community physicians who have been granted privileges and will also orient new faculty and introduce the physician relations program and it's expectations.

As the hospital provides more direction on growth of specific service lines, we are ready to deliver specific messages to the referring audience to drive referrals to those areas.

Wayne Sensor
CEO
CHRISTUS Schumpert Health System
Shreveport, LA

(Editor's note: In mid-2004, Sensor assumed the CEO post for Alegent Health in Omaha, NE.)

What were some market conditions that led you to implement a physician relations strategy?

Things we used to take for granted that we did for and with our physicians aren't allowed anymore. And as physicians scramble to supplant their shrinking revenue, they're participating in joint ventures and carve-outs that shift revenue from hospitals. These factors are polarizing relationships between hospitals and physicians. The relationship sales model can very much help to bring us back together.

The primary driver for our physician strategy was a desire to increase market share. While we wanted to retain the referral base we had, we needed to grow targeted volumes. We evaluated the experience and success that for-profit hospitals and specialty services, such as rehabilitation and behavioral health, had with a formal sales approach. We wanted a referral development model that would fit our environment and medical staff culture while also generating the desired referral results. We thought and were convinced that implementing a model like this would drive some incremental volume and market share into our hospital. From our vantage point, it is the single most significant physician relations strategy that we've developed in the last three years.

How did you go about making your senior leadership team comfortable with a sales-oriented strategy?

Once my VP of Marketing and Planning and I bought off on the concept, we spent a lot of time on the front end educating the senior leadership team as to the value that sales could bring to the organization. I would say freely that we convinced some but not all; I made a decision to move forward and sort of bring the others along by proving the results.

How have you measured success because of your efforts?

We measure results in two different ways. There's a quantitative piece and a bit of a qualitative piece. Part of making this model successful is you must be clear about what you're going to measure and how you're going to measure it to prove the efficacy of the investment. What we track are referrals from new sources, doctors who weren't using our hospital at all, and so we are targeting them for a particular service or services and we're tracking new business from them.

We also measure increases from existing referring physicians. We trend very tightly and carefully both up and down trends from doctors. We're looking, of course, to grow the business from new as well as existing physicians. A caveat of that is sometimes from an existing physician that's an existing service line they're referring to. For example, a physician that may have been sending us the general medicine inpatients already, we may extend the rehabilitation service to that physician and now you start to see referrals to our rehabilitation programs.

Additionally, we track new referrals by geographic area. We track by ZIP code and know what the referral patterns are from that ZIP code, as opposed to doctor. We may target that particular community, so we'll also track referrals in that manner from geography.

How does tracking help the organization keep better tabs on things and be able to make adjustments?

I never cease to be amazed that, if you're not tracking it and watching it carefully, physicians who are heavy users to the hospital will fall off and nobody knows. It's a matter of you've got a lot of physicians, you've got a lot of volume, a lot of different programs and services, that if you don't have that discipline it will take you six months to figure out that somebody has an issue with the hospital and has stopped using you. Or conversely, somebody who has started to use your hospital substantially or refer for services and you don't take an opportunity to acknowledge that.

You have to be a little careful because a week doesn't make a trend but it gives us as an organization a chance to keep its eye expressly on the ball. And the translation is to make adjustments: Does the CEO need to make a sales call on that person or, on the happy side, does the CEO need to jot this physician a note? When I see the doctor in the surgeon's lounge, it blows him away if I say, 'I've noticed you've referred 10 patients to us in the last two months. Thank you for your trust.'

Why have you, as a CEO, made it a point to be involved in the program?

I've learned a lot from my sales force. They are the eyes and ears for the CEO to keep in touch with those relationships and for me to personally give them sound bites about things that are going on so they can extend my message into the marketplace. They also become my extension into the marketplace, allowing me more visibility and options to meet with physicians than if I do this by myself. If we've got anything of significance going on that's going to affect my medical staff, my sales force always knows before it's implemented.

Before we implemented this effort here, I would have readily said I was very much in touch with our key physicians and that I knew what was going on in the market. It's amazing—it's *amazing*—what the sales force learns when they build relationships with the physician in the office, make calls that bring value and develop trust around this relationship. I'm always interested to attend the sales meeting to understand that they picked up market intelligence about a new service being developed, that a new competitor is entering the market, or an opportunity is uncovered—we've had some great leads about opportunities to grow our business that was revealed in a sales call to one of our sales team.

What would you do differently next time—in planning, execution or evaluation?

There are two lessons learned that stick with us. One is, you've got to have the right leader of the sales initiative—a balance between someone who has analytical skills, can make sense of the data and direct the effort and someone who is a pure salesperson and is comfortable asking for business.
We learned that we tipped the scale a little bit toward the analytical end and didn't see the project or initiative grow and nurture the way we hoped and we had to make a leadership change. By not carefully

understanding the competencies and the right profile, that made our program hiccup and start a little slowly.

What we learned upon our implementation, there are many silos—and people protect their data. It requires in many cases that Leadership tear down the silos. Also, a lot of times the data simply doesn't exist or doesn't exist in a format that's useful for sales.

The other thing that I suspect is almost universally applicable is data, data, data. I thought we had decent data systems and that it would be readily available to feed our sales efforts-because without it, you're blind. Without it, you don't know where you're getting your business, for what services, from whom and therefore how to direct your sales effort.

For example, we have a well-developed hospitalist program at our institution. That means an outlying primary care physician can refer to one of our hospitalists who will admit the patient. Our data system prior to sales being implemented would have shown the admission as the hospitalist, rather than from the referring physician. We asked the questions but our information system didn't capture who that other physician was. When you stripped it off and tried to garner where those patients were coming from, we found hundreds of admissions relating to our hospitalists, which is absolutely irrelevant.

We had to go back and in some cases capture the right data points. In many cases, we had to reformat or build reports that more effectively supported the sales effort. That took us some time and energy. I would caution everyone: Don't underestimate the importance of data to focus your sales effort, but know that it will also take some time and attention on the front end.

What are the expectations for the representative when they call on a physician?

These people schedule formal appointments with a physician—they don't ever walk in unexpected. When they get there, they're very clear about what this practice looks like. We've profiled it and know a great deal about the practice, and we're bringing something of value to the doctor. This is not donuts or dinner. This is not, "How are you doing, I'd like your business.'

This is, we're walking into a GYN's office and we're going to introduce him to the availability of our new GYN oncological surgeon who is available for both phone consults and certainly live consults on difficult patients. He's here to help you, Dr. GYN.

These are not casual conversations. These are 10-minute focused value that we bring to that physician. Frequently, the doctor will make it 45 minutes because they're so excited that somebody's brought something of measurable value. Often, you'll open up the dike and they'll tell you all kinds of things and give you all kinds of opportunities.

What are some must-haves from your perspective, or advice for your peers?

A physician relations program is an exceptionally effective method to build volume and strengthen relationships. We've been slow to recognize and realize that the for-profits and, particularly, the niche providers have been doing this for years. To apply that in other settings can build business and can indeed strengthen relationships.

Front-end design is exceptionally important. If you don't have the expertise, solicit the help of someone who does.

Involvement of Leadership is critical. If you can't get it, it will not be successful. Data will determine whether you're shooting a shotgun or a rifle. Only with data can you focus the sales effort in the right direction so they spend their time wisely and effectively.

How has the use of outside consultants helped you with program implementation?

It is absolutely critical that there be substantial time and energy spent on the front end to design the process. How are you going to organize it? How does it relate back to strategy? How does the leader plug in with the rest of the senior leadership team? What metrics are you going to measure? What kind of model are you going to use?

I made a very conscious decision when we began looking at the development of a physician sales model to use outside resources. My reason for that was that there were exactly two of us on the senior leadership team—myself and one other—that had knowledge of a formalized sales approach. We did not feel like, based on that assessment, that we had the horsepower to build this thing.

We didn't have the expertise and I thought the learning curve was going to be too long. We chose consciously to use an outside resource to build it. They helped with the business plan, job descriptions and they helped the selection of the final leader for the sales effort. They did some training for us. I believe that was critical in the success of our sales effort. It would have taken us a year and a half to bring the thing up and I think the probability of success would have been far less.

Nancy Dugas
Healthcare Consultant
Strategy and Business Development
Shreveport, LA

(Dugas formerly was Vice President, Strategy for CHRISTUS Schumpert Health System in Shreveport, LA.)

What have you gained by using a physician relations strategy in your prior position?

The organization saw incremental growth in designated services, new physician referral sources, strengthened relationships with existing physicians and branching off into employer strategies concurrently. Its cancer treatment center visits increased 23 percent in the first year of the program and saw a sustained increase in the second year; the accumulated increase is now 29 percent.

There have been more than 100 new referrals from primary care providers. Twenty-seven new physicians are now referring to the region. There are 16,000 covered lives in the M.D. Anderson Physicians Network. _CHRISTUS_ opened new markets in the fringe of its tertiary market.

What would you do differently next time—in planning, execution or evaluation?

Hire the right director. We only had one candidate that qualified initially, so we took our chances and he lasted fewer than 90 days. Also, determine who is on board in Senior Leadership.

What ongoing challenges do you face with your program?

Continuing the momentum, maintaining and succeeding the gain. Keeping the sales force energized.

Going forward, how do you intend to grow or reshape your program?

The organization recently took operational responsibility for urgent care clinics and occupational health—all to be used to support the primary care physician network and strengthen access points. These areas report to the sales director. The vision is to have all these areas relate to Business Development, supported by Sales.

Donna Teach
Vice President, Marketing and Public Relations
Columbus Children's Hospital
Columbus, OH

How did you move your program forward?

The first thing I did was make sure I had a very strong champion who believed in this program. In our case, that was our medical director; he continues to be one of the strongest advocates of this program. He served as our partner in having these discussions that involved our CEO, our president and COO, Chief Nursing Officer, Chief Financial Officer, Managed Care—all of our administrative functions and our clinical functions, as well—to really determine what we want to get out of the program.

We brought into that session a white paper overview to benchmark other programs and used that to show and aid the discussion about what do we and don't want this program to be. Our development cycle for the whole program from the time we came up with the program to when we had the liaisons in the field was 12 months. I think we needed every bit of that to really build the program correctly.

How did you involve Leadership in the planning process?

My first phase was doing benchmarking, did my homework, developed a business case, really educated myself and did some stakeholder interviews. Then, probably within the first 60 days we were having these discussions with Senior Leadership. It didn't take long to reach consensus once we got the right people around the table, but these were very important discussions to have.

It takes a balance of opinion to make this happen. Some people in the organization really viewed this as a key element of our quality initiatives. They felt the most important thing this program was going to do was enhance communication with our referring physicians and our medical staff. Others at the table saw the financial potential.

What role have performance measures played in your strategy?

The development of competency documents was really the bringing to life for the sales team of these goals and expectations. Our competency document is really the lifeblood of our program for our liaisons. They are a series of expectations—measurable, quantifiable, defined expectations—that map out for the liaisons exactly what is expected of them. Their performance and their compensation is directly linked to their performance on these targeted competencies.

I find, again, when talking with peers, that's the biggest challenge. I think you reap what you sow: If you give people clear direction and hold them clearly accountable and they know what's expected of them, generally that motivates salespeople—they're very goal-driven people generally. That strategy has worked very well for us.

How do your representatives handle issue resolution?

When liaisons and salespeople go out, they are going to encounter problems in the field; that's part of their job. Often, that's a barrier to building a further relationship that's going to result in referrals. You have two choices: Either you're going to hire and use your liaisons as problem-solvers, which in my opinion is not what you want them to do. You're not paying your salespeople to be out there solving problems.

You need an infrastructure inside the organization to which those salespeople can bring those issues—basically an issue resolution process where you have organizational accountability to help address issues brought in from the liaisons. I want them to identify the problems and bring them to the right person; the organization needs to hold that person accountable for addressing those issues or problems. We want the liaison to do the follow-up.

Our issue resolution process at Children's is very robust. We have a very structured process that actually is led by our medical director and chief operating officer. They see every issue that comes in from the field. They triage them and determine who's the accountable party. We have very strong rigor around how those issues are dealt with and loaded into a database so we can track them and learn from them.

The salesperson may have to earn their spurs with some practices. If the practice feels the liaison doesn't have the backing of the organization, it damages their credibility. They don't view the liaison as strongly as they could.

Imagine you send a salesperson out in the field, the practice raises an issue and 24 hours later they get a call from the chief of that department. That does two things: It sends a very strong customer-service message, but it also positions your salesperson as someone who is a very credible, valuable source within the organization.

It's the number-one thing we hear from the doctors out there that they really, really value. They feel those liaisons are advocates for them and that their voice is heard within the organization.

What criteria do you set in the hiring process?

We do two types of interviewing. We interview for organization fit and we interview for sales skills. I would hire a salesperson who has little to no healthcare knowledge long before I will hire a very strong healthcare person who has little to no sales background. We feel pretty strongly that you can learn healthcare—although we've always ended up hiring people with healthcare sales experience—but you really want to hire for sales skills first.

I don't want to stereotype clinical folks, but generally folks go into clinical care because they like to help people and solve problems. That's not what you want your salesperson to do. You want your salesperson to position, influence choice and be incentivized along sales-driven goals—such as generating new business and changing people's referral patterns. That's a different skill set.

How is your interview process structured?

We do behaviorally based interviewing with them. We actually do role-playing with them and look for certain characteristics in their presentation style. We have an outside party that specializes in this type of interviewing that does this with us to assess their strength and sales skills.

There are three tiers to it. I interview first for organizational fit and basic sales skills. We put them through the behaviorally based sales interview with the external party. The third phase is with the internal stakeholders. I won't hire a salesperson who doesn't pass by my medical director.

How do you get the internal team on board with your strategy?

You have to market your program internally—really, internally is most important. People have to understand who the representatives are. You've got to help them be supported inside the organization. Our medical director was our communication arm. We did over 25 presentations to help the organization understand why we were doing this. We generate quarterly reports and communicate within the organization what the program is doing.

In the launch phase, it's so important to let people know why you're doing this, what is it, what value is it to them internally and to really position the representatives as a valued resource within the organization. Then you need to continue to communicate—very important. Some people don't understand what sales is. Everybody has a different impression about what they think it is. It's not necessarily always viewed as a positive thing.

Has this kind of communication had an effect on how the program has been received externally?

Absolutely. It's huge. You're paying someone to bring issues to light out in the market and that can be perceived as not necessarily a positive thing internally. It was very important, when the liaisons brought these issues internally and we started this issue resolution process that involves our medical director and chief operating officer and president, that people thought this was a good thing. It also was important when they called these practices back that this was perceived as a positive.

That in fact has been the case for us because it's really helped our operational leads to build relationships with our referral sources. What we've seen over time is that when physicians had issues they might have called the liaisons first, but now they actually have a contact in the department they know and can call. Operational folks love that and really value that. They want to deal with their own customers.

What didn't go as well as you thought it would?

Our ROI models are sort of a perpetual work in progress for us and other healthcare organizations. I think everybody does it a little bit differently. Initially, we did not focus as much on how we were going to measure the ROI. It was identified obviously as a key area and we had metrics in place that we were going to track. I think it's very difficult to build a global ROI model for a sales function, because there's so much cause and effect.

You can say, overall our referral business went up three percent this year and there's millions of dollars associated with that—what percentage of that money was as a result of the sales function? Building global ROI models is very challenging. We have developed a variety of financial models that focus more at the product-line level to demonstrate financial and organizational and financial impact.

For example, we actually sell lab contracts in partnership with our reference laboratory service here at Children's. That is new revenue in the door. There is no question that that is a direct result of the liaison function. That's an example of a very focused, targeted direct cause-and-effect ROI.

There are more macro models we do look at that have less direct cause and effect. For example, we target certain geographic counties over the course of the year. We track referrals coming out of that county—did they go up, did they go down? That's more of a macro model. We know we've impacted that, but it's hard to say. Say we had a very heavy or light flu season. Well, that influences referrals. There are a lot of things that can help or hurt referral business that may be outside the control of the sales function.

You need to reach agreement with your chief financial officer about how they want to measure this.

What have you gained by using a physician relations strategy?

When successfully implemented, an effective physician relations strategy will pay off through both short-term and long-term returns. In the short term, our organization benefits from increased referrals and physician satisfaction. The long-term benefits, specifically enhanced physician loyalty and retention, are truly priceless. It's difficult to place a dollar value on satisfied physicians but I would prefer this qualitative value to counting the dollar and cents losses associated from a disenfranchised member of our medical staff or the loss of a referring physician.

What measurable results can you report?

Organizationally, our most important focus is on the enhanced clinical quality that results from more effective communication with physicians. For example, the enhancements to clinical care and safety realized through our computerized order entry system are extensive. Within Marketing, our results are measured through positive attitudinal changes and enhanced referral patterns. We conduct annual physician satisfaction surveys with our liaison function as well as a financial audit of our sales efforts. These are regularly reported to our administrative team.

What would you do differently next time—in planning, execution or evaluation?

I can honestly say I wouldn't change too many things about the implementation of our physician relations strategy. The keys to success are organizational consensus on goals and direction, clear physician championing and lots of patience!

What are some must-haves from your perspective, or advice for your peers?

Regarding physician sales, I'm a strong believer in hiring for sales talent before product knowledge. I see many unsuccessful programs where the sales representative becomes the "problem solver," spending time in the office dealing with issues instead of being in the field seeing doctors. This appears to be an intrinsic characteristic and problem for many caregivers who enter sales. I seek physician sales representatives who know how to build strong problem-solving relationships within the hospital so they can focus their time in the field.

Other must-haves for sales programs include a clear and accountable model for issue resolution. When sales representatives are presented with a problem or concern from a physician there must be a clear internal process for responding to that issue in a timely manner. We spent months building our issue resolution model and it's been a key to success for our program.

Going forward, how do you intend to grow or reshape your program?

Our next step at Columbus Children's is expanding our successful regional model to a multi-state focus. We are adding liaisons to sell specific niche services we offer, such as congenital heart surgery, that are unique in the Midwest. This will open an exciting new chapter for us.

Kathy Dean
Associate Vice President, Marketing
Geisinger Health System
Danville, PA

What measurable results can you report?

Number one, we're getting clear results and have seen referrals increase. A physician had sent us 44 referrals the first half of the year. We started making calls on him in May 2003 and we saw 84 referrals the second half of the year.

We've also been able to broaden our reach for our high-end services—our tertiary and quaternary services. Those are all referral-based and we can do it through the physician liaison program, reaching into areas our advertising doesn't reach. These physicians are in remote or rural areas and need to send their patients out of the area for care. Our goal is to say, "We'd like you to send them to us."

What didn't go the way you thought it would? What would you change in hindsight?

I think having a good database to start with would have been a good thing to do. We have struggled way too long with trying to get a handle on who is actually out in our area and verifying who they are. Even now, we've transferred this database. We've tried to clean it up as much as we could by cross-referencing it electronically with existing records. But I finally said, "We have got to get this right and we have to know it's right." We have a temporary employee who is calling every physician office and verifying this information.

What ongoing challenges do you face with your program?

The biggest thing we still struggle with is how much is too much communication with the liaisons. It's a fine line to walk between keeping them informed of everything that's going on and getting them comfortable with new services and new doctors, changes in a service line and making sure they're out on the road. It's really easy to get them sucked into too many internal meetings. It's something I fight every month. I'm looking at it again—do we really need all these meetings and how can we schedule them so they're at a time that's convenient for the liaisons and not in the middle of prime selling time?

What are some must-haves for a program?

I think you need an operations champion, someone who understands the value of the program and will help to change the culture to make it open to suggestions from the external side. I was lucky: At the same time that we were retooling this program and knew where we wanted to go with it in Marketing, the Chief Administrative Officer started a referring physician relationship task force. It pulled in some of the key doctors internally and helped generate a focused approach in relationships with referring physicians.

Going forward, how do you intend to grow or reshape your program?

More of the same. This year we're looking at quantity of visits. Next year, we're looking at quality of visits—how can we get the face time with the doctor—and that's what we'll be measuring. We'll be really looking at measurements we're doing on a consistent basis and confirming that the people out there are doing what they say they're doing.

Lynne Meyers
Vice President, Planning, Marketing & Business Development
Montgomery General Hospital
Olney, MD

What measurable results can you report?

Our program is new, so there are no tangible wins such as X number of new physicians or new admissions. What I can describe is physician groups who were planning on dropping their privileges, changing their minds after being visited by our liaison and being informed about some of our up-and-coming programs. Also, we've had a tremendous number of "leads" where doors have been opened for us to engage in detailed conversations with large groups who were potentially interested in coming to our hospital.

What would you do differently next time—in planning, execution or evaluation?

We're struggling with the "art" of closing the deal. We're doing well in terms of finding leads, opening doors and having nice conversations with physicians. I wish we had spent more time thinking through how to take the next step and make it incredibly easy for physicians to come on board.

What are some must-haves from your perspective, or advice for your peers?

1) Hire someone with a strong sales background! Chances are you can teach someone about "hospital stuff." I don't think it's as easy to teach someone about sales.
2) Be very specific about how you want to approach your existing medical staff; create segments such as "CEO's inner circle," top admitters, occasional admitters, etc.
3) Work to create a good relationship between your marketing department and physician liaison(s).

Lyle D. Green, MBA, CHE
Assistant Vice President for Referral Development
University of Texas M.D. Anderson Cancer Center
Houston, TX

What have you gained by using a physician relations strategy?

At the M. D. Anderson Cancer Center, we have gained several things:

Our ability to establish relationships with community physicians has grown from approximately 500 per year in 1996 to over 3,750 in 2003. This is primarily due to the growth of program resources during that timeframe.

We have created significant internal awareness for the value and importance of establishing and maintaining strong relationships with community and referring physicians. This has been the result of significant time and effort spent in discussions, meetings, and presentations across the organization describing the physician referral base (e.g., who they are, where they practice, where they refer to, what their needs and expectations are with regards to their interactions with M. D. Anderson).

What measurable results can you report?

Physician referral activity has increased by approximately 21 percent from fiscal year 1997 to fiscal year 2003, while new patient registration activity from physician referrals has increased approximately 19 percent during the same time period.

Referring Physician Satisfaction scores have improved significantly. M. D. Anderson has conducted an ongoing satisfaction survey process since March 2000. "Top-Two Box" scores for "Overall Satisfaction" have increased from 72 percent in fiscal year 2000 to 80.3 percent by the end of fiscal year 2003.

M. D. Anderson's physician reputational score in the annual *U.S. News and World Report* "Best Hospital Rankings" has exceeded 70 in three of the past four years (2000, 2003, and 2003). At no other time since the inception of the best hospital rankings has the M. D. Anderson physician reputational score exceeded 70. In each of those three years, M. D. Anderson has been named the nation's number-one cancer center.

The Oncology Roundtable of the Advisory Board Company recognized the M. D. Anderson Physician Relations program as a best practice during its 2001 Oncology Leadership Agenda: Creating an Exceptional Cancer Enterprise.

M. D. Anderson's *Guide for Referring Physicians* publication won a bronze award for Physician Referral Program in Healthcare Marketing Report's Nineteenth Annual Healthcare Advertising Awards program (2002).

What would you do differently next time—in planning, execution or evaluation?

- Conduct additional in-depth research with referring physicians on the perceived value and expectations for service and support that can be provided by physician liaison/a physician relations program.
- Conduct more and regular training for staff members. Create a true staff development program for physician liaison staff.
- Continually review the skill mix of physician liaison staff, taking into consideration the need and value for recruitment of clinical, non-clinical, and/or experience in sales, marketing, and/or customer service.
- Develop and implement a more robust contact/relationship management system with appropriate interfaces to hospital information systems.

What are some must-haves from your perspective, or advice for your peers?

- Have support from organizational leadership, internal faculty and staff.
- Be able to demonstrate the value of the physician relations/liaison role to the organization.

- Recognize the community physician as a primary customer of the organization.
- Leverage technology and the Internet to the greatest extent possible.
- Be able to obtain the necessary data and information, and have the ability to translate this into knowledge that reflects the needs and expectations of the referring physician.
- Have a process for obtaining continuous feedback from referring physicians about what is working well and what is not working well, and the ability to translate this into recommendations for process and operations improvement that supports referral interactions with community physicians.
- Understand that this does not happen overnight—be patient with the process.
- And, above all, maintain your sense of humor!

What ongoing challenges do you face with your program?

- Providing direct contact/relationship management support to approximately 8,000 to 10,000 referring physicians nationwide with limited resources.
- Developing a solid process to maintain current demographic (address/contact) information for our referring physicians.
- Working within hospital operations to streamline the new patient referral process for physician-referred patients.
- Developing solutions to facilitate and improve physician-to-physician communications.

Going forward, how do you intend to grow or reshape your program?

Our program has evolved gradually and incrementally over the years; I do not foresee this approach changing in the near term. We are currently recruiting for a newly created liaison role to provide focus on pediatric oncology referrals.

Longer term, I see more emphasis to move referring physician interactions (e.g., referral process, insurance authorization, follow-up communications) to the Internet to improve efficiency and cost-effectiveness of those processes.

Our program is becoming more directly engaged in hospital operations and process improvement efforts. While we have historically collaborated closely with staff in hospital operations in this area, we have, within the past two years taken on more of a leadership role in conducting processes aimed at developing solutions to improve aspects of the new patient referral process. We have also taken on the role of "process owner" for a major information system component of the referring physician follow-up communications process.

Russ Sesto
Physician Liaison Manager
University of Wisconsin and Health Services
Madison, WI

What have you gained by using a physician relations strategy?

The liaison program has resulted in better relationships with not only our referring physicians, but also the internal physicians, Administration and Leadership.

Key areas of enhancement include:

- Improved communication with internal and external physicians, nurses, payors, administrators, clinic managers, referral coordinators
- Better and faster methods for handling referral concerns. These generally involve communication issues such as assisting with appointment schedule, discharge records and clinic records.
- Assistance for our referring physicians/staff in facilitating connections with the right resources.
- The ability to provide physicians with a greater knowledge of specialty/clinical services, including an ability to provide a faster and greater knowledge of new services, protocols and new specialists.
- Creating opportunities for physician site visits (opportunity to see UWHC and meet physician) and providing educational programs at their location or ours.

Beyond the routine functions, the program has provided market intelligence, which helps our Leadership determine how to grow and defend our strategic position and meet the hospital's goals.

What measurable results can you report?

Our measurements include both a report of liaison activity as well as revenue and volume numbers, such as:

- Number of physicians we meet with monthly
- Inpatient and outpatient data by market

- Revenue by market
- Increase in positive impressions by physician leaders, physician and Senior Leadership within UWHC, as well as external to the organization

What would you do differently next time—in planning, execution or evaluation?

In hindsight, there are two areas where I believe the physician liaison program should have had more integration. The first is to tie the program into our call center program. The second area is to get more involved and offer more about the program to our new doctors.

What are some must-haves from your perspective, or advice for your peers?

- Get Leadership buy-in and support of the program.
- Work closely with Outreach and Marketing departments.
- Have a strong decision support staff to run numbers and then create a reliable physician database and a reporting database. Use one database, updated regularly, for referring physicians.
- Hire good staff and take the time to train them on your facility. Train routinely on areas that are needed to keep them successful.
- Have an adequate budget.
- Stay credible with internal and external customers/physicians/payors.

What ongoing challenges do you face with your program?

- Money/budget issues
- Getting accurate data you can rely on
- Contracting issues

- Balancing meeting the needs of the system and the needs of individual physicians or programs
- Growing and defending markets
- Prioritizing service lines

Going forward, how do you intend to grow or reshape your program?

We want to grow the program by having the manager do less roadwork and more internal activities. However, I believe the manager needs to be involved in some fieldwork and cannot be 100 percent behind the desk.

Gail Callandrillo
Vice President, Planning & Market Research
The Valley Hospital
Ridgewood, NJ

What measurable results can you report?

Volume to the Same Day Surgery Center, improved satisfaction with hospital services and high satisfaction with the program (4.54 of a possible 5).

What are some must-haves from your perspective, or advice for your peers?

Absolute support from the top, close communication with the medical staff leaders, absolute trust with the individual(s), results where possible. Nothing breeds success like success. When you can get those quick wins, go for it. Most of the issues are operational and systemic in nature and are going to take some time. Keep the momentum going with the quick wins and you'll know what those are when you come across them.

What ongoing challenges do you face with your program?

Increasing pressures on physicians that we cannot assist with, such as malpractice, managed care or a loss of income. Other challenges include keeping your physicians happy to reduce the threat of competitive action (e.g., investing in a surgi-center).

Beverly Miller
Director, Physician Relations
The Valley Hospital
Ridgewood, NJ

What have you gained by using a physician relations strategy?

Doctors and their office staff really appreciate the effort and expense that the hospital is willing to incur to have me out on the road. I am able to keep initiatives important to physicians on the front burner, whereas otherwise they fall back to the bottom of the pile.

What measurable results can you report?

- Contact people throughout the organization have addressed over 650 issues since program inception.
- Relationships with office managers have improved with quarterly OM meetings and the formation of a several-member office manager advisory board.

- 180 Valley Health System leaders have submitted and implemented their own physician satisfaction ideas.
- A strategy for new physicians has been developed along with a "Resource Guide" for new physicians to share with their staff.

What are some must-haves from your perspective, or advice for your peers?

- *Always* honor confidentiality with physicians—it is tempting to vary from this, *but don't!*
- Train your contact people in advance how to handle issue resolution. We still have some problems with defensiveness; this is a hard habit to break.
- You need a boss who can brainstorm and think out of the box. I'm fortunate to have this.
- Work closely with your medical staff leadership and department directors. They can be your best allies (or, in some cases, your biggest challenge).

What ongoing challenges do you face with your program?

Each month that goes by it is more and more difficult to keep up with my visits. I don't get involved in "issue solving," but I do get involved in developing strategies for larger system fixes and program strategy. This involvement seems to be logarithmic as more and more people are now calling me for advice. I have been quite visible since I've been doing presentations at our one- and two-day leadership institutes and I think this is driving some of the requests for consultation. My involvement has driven some important changes and program growth, so I feel that I need to stay involved, but it saps my time.

Conclusion

There's nothing like living through an experience to really understand—and appreciate—the effort that's involved. As we review the stories in the special section of these wise and occasionally battered experts who are implementing great programs, there are some common threads. Their words of wisdom and our experiences with clients across the country resound with the need to:

1. *Pay attention to the people part of the program.* In order to have a good physician relations program, you need the right staff in the right positions. They need to know what's expected of them and have the tenacity to persist in attaining the goals. Give them the training they need to be successful. As you develop or re-tool your program, pay attention to making sure you know what you want the person to do; hire for that focus and give them the freedom and support to their obligations.

2. *Be strategic—take the time to make a plan and do it right.* Rely on the data combined with intuitive resources of the leadership team to define the path. You need clarity in your goals and direction. Too many "nice to do" projects will de-rail the central focus unless you clearly articulate your purpose.

3. *Never underestimate the need for internal integration and support.* Every single successful program leader talks about the need for support of Senior Leadership. Beyond Leadership buy-in, develop a mechanism for operational responsiveness to problems, communication and access issues to ensure you can deliver on the promise.

4. *Communicate—over and over again.* There's a compelling need to:

   a) Keep messages fresh and consistent for the external referring physicians.
   b) Keep the physician relations team informed regarding internal updates.
   c) Keep the key internal stakeholders aware of field intelligence.

5. *Innovate and try new approaches.* It's the thing that will set your program apart. Steer clear of the "vendor row" in the physician's waiting room by offering that special sizzle that only a physician relations person can provide.

We can't stress it enough: There are many right ways to build a physician relations program. The key to find the one right for you is to look at your organization and its current medical staff relationships. Ask yourself and your team, "What can it offer physicians in a competitive environment?"

Give yourself and your team the permission and the freedom to make some mistakes along the way. You'll learn more from the mistakes you make from anything else.

Continue to validate the wisdom of those you work with—the doctors who trust you enough to send a referral in your direction, and the Leadership who continue to provide you with the resources to do it well.

Thanks for the opportunity to share our thoughts. Moving forward, the field of physician relations will continue to evolve. We look forward to participating in that journey and invite you to join us on the ride!

# # #